What Is Wrong With ME

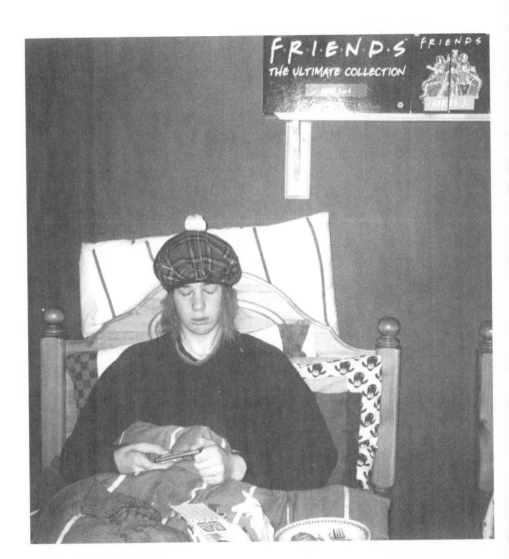

What Is Wrong With ME

A Case of childhood Myalgic Encephalomyelitis

The Illness and the Controversy

Merryn Fergusson

The Grimsay Press

The Grimsay Press
an imprint of
Zeticula Ltd
The Roan
Kilkerran
KA19 8LS
Scotland.

http://www.thegrimsaypress.co.uk
admin@thegrimsaypress.co.uk

First published 2012.

Text © Merryn Fergusson 2012

Cover design © David McNeill 2012

ISBN-13 978-1-84530-126-2

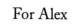
For Alex

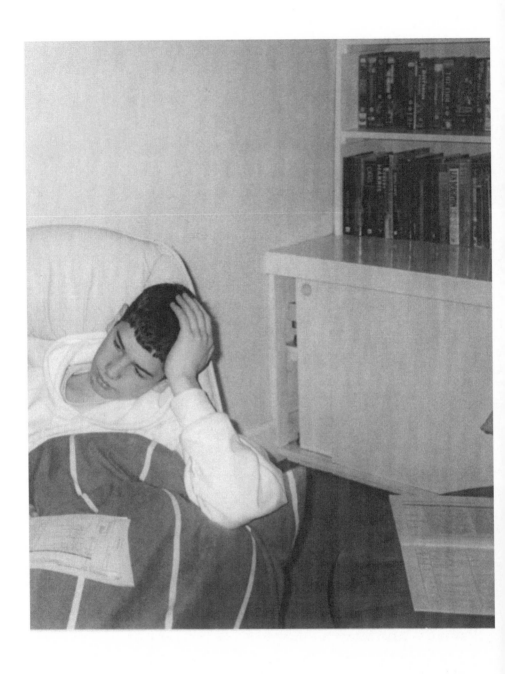

Acknowledgements

I would like to thank the following people for their help and encouragement during the seven years that it has taken to write this book.

My childhood friend Joy Pemberton-Piggot spent hours proofreading and was the first to remark that "I had no idea that ME was like that", which spurred me on.

My fellow physiotherapist and lifelong friend Jane Bignell spent many hours researching past papers on ME with me and never allowed me to give up. In 2007 her own son developed ME, from which he is finally on the road to recovery.

Debra Hall, a creative writer and an inspirational mentor, was a hard and valued task master. Danny Aston wrote a most professional critique for me when I tried for a second time to get published.

Miranda Bowles, Cathy Agnew and Sheila Butler gave generously of their time and their advice.

Before I had a computer Moira Duncan, who suffers from Multiple Sclerosis, looked over the original version and typed it out for me.

I sent the second draft to my mother, Diana Barthold, who, rightly, because I was still so angry by the fate suffered by ME patients that I was unable to write sufficiently dispassionately, suggested that I wait a couple of years.

In 2011 I sent the third manuscript to Sir Charles Fergusson, who wrote "What an awful ordeal you all had with Chris' ME. 'The half was not told me' (1 Kings 2 vii). *That,* felt by me, possibly justifies pushing ahead with your book." He advised that I contact the Writer's Workshop and as a result Claire Gillman's appraisal persuaded me to virtually re-write the book. Through Charles I found a publisher.

I am also grateful to my colleagues at FASIC, the sports injury clinic at Edinburgh University, for their friendship.

This is my chance to thank all those who helped Chris throughout the time that he was housebound. Whether or not you are mentioned in the story, you know who you are.

However, the Thursday boys and Danny Maguire merit a special mention. The young school boys were never prompted to visit Chris every week, but they became, although they could not have known it, Chris' life savers. When no treatment is available and you are suffering from an unrecognised illness, the endorsement of your friends is of paramount importance.

I am grateful for the understanding and support that Chris received from the Headmaster and Staff of Stewart Melville College.

No book about childhood ME would be complete without mentioning Dr Nigel Speight. He features in Chris' story, but there are thousands of people who are indebted to this good, kind, dedicated and courageous doctor. Dr Speight will probably never receive any formal recognition. He is available to all ME sufferers, gives talks around the world and says that he is unable to understand why he is a lone voice.

Should this book realise any profits they will be donated to bio-medical research into ME in Scotland. All ME sufferers have reason to be grateful to Dr Vance Spence, Dr Neil Abbot and their colleagues for their dedication and skilled work at ME Research UK in Perth.

Merryn Fergusson
August, 2012

Contents

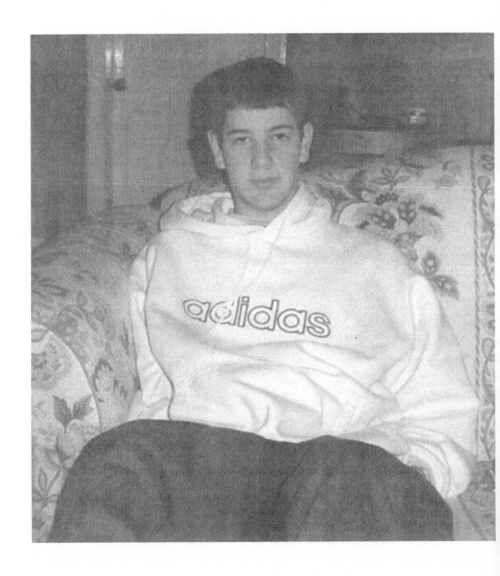

Introduction

Our teenage son, Chris, was diagnosed with Myalgic Encephalomyelitis (ME) when, after three years of increasing ill-health, he became bed-ridden. ME is the most common cause of long-term sickness absence from school, rating higher than cancer, yet because of a lack of knowledge these children are neglected and forgotten.

The average bout of ME lasts for four and a half years and most children contract it at around the age of twelve when they are moving into secondary education. The longevity and nature of the illness and the age at which it strikes leaves children isolated from their peers. It also severely compromises their academic and sporting education and their social development.

Despite the fact that nine thousand families in UK have a child with ME, research has been scarce. This lack of commitment is mainly owing to the controversy between physicians and psychiatrists regarding the condition. Physicians maintain that ME is a physical illness and psychiatrists maintain that ME is a mental condition. The lack of a clear identity for the disease causes confusion in the medical profession and therefore among the public.

While there is this dilemma children continue to suffer and are destined to remain shadows unnoticed by society. They are condemned to an illness in which disbelief, lack of care and minimal investigations are commonplace, and in which they may face actual or threatened removal from their homes.

This story could be said to describe Chris' battle with ME, but a battle infers an active involvement with a recognisable enemy. In reality ME is more like a siege, where the patient passively endures everything his unseen foe hurls at him without knowing when, or if, it will cease.

During his illness Chris was unable to read, watch films, or enjoy the company of his friends, all the while feeling as if he was being poisoned.

He eventually emerged from his bedroom prison and had to learn belatedly how to adjust to the role of a teenager. As the first stirrings of recovery began to emerge, every advance towards regaining his health reinforced Chris' resolve never to waste a second of any day that he was well enough to enjoy. Now that he no longer feels the stigma of ME, and so as to speak for other sufferers, he has allowed me to tell his story.

1986

"But alas to make me
The fixed figure for the time of scorn
To point his slow and moving finger at."

John Milton

1986 was a significant year in the turbulent history of ME. In 1986 Dr Melvin Ramsay wrote that patients with Myalgic Encephalomyelitis would no longer have to dread their doctors telling them that 'all your tests are clear, therefore there is nothing the matter with you'.

Dr Ramsay had been the consultant in infectious diseases at the Royal Free hospital in London in 1955 when a major epidemic of Myalgic Encephalomyelitis had struck. At that time the mysterious illness, which forced the hospital to close because so many of its staff were affected, had been labelled simply the Royal Free disease, but once Dr Ramsay and his colleagues had recorded their investigations and presented them to the medical world it had been given the name Myalgic Encephalo-Myelitis.

When the unknown disease broke out in the Royal Free Hospital epidemics of serious illnesses were still occurring regularly. Treatments were only then emerging that would eventually largely eradicate polio, whooping cough, measles, scarlet fever, and diphtheria, all of which are potentially fatal. These diseases are highly contagious, they generate a great deal of fear, and elaborate precautions were taken to prevent them spreading. The patient was isolated and put in quarantine, they were carefully nursed, and they had a long convalescence. It was a time when the concept of new diseases was not met with scepticism. Indeed, new diseases such as Legionnaire's disease, Ebola virus and AIDS were yet to arrive.

When ME appears in the general run of medicine the onset is similar to that of an epidemic. It can start as an alarming attack of acute vertigo, or as a respiratory tract infection, or gastro-enteritis with nausea and vomiting. Instead of the expected recovery, the patient is dogged by a profound fatigue accompanied by a variety of symptoms and a general sense of 'feeling awful'. All cases run a low-grade fever which usually subsides in a week, then patients are left with symptoms in the muscles, the circulation, and the brain. Muscles fatigue after activity, taking three or more days to recover their normal power, and in severe cases may have twitchings, spasms and be acutely tender to touch. Circulation is impaired, with the patient having cold extremities, a sensitivity to changes of temperature, and an ashen-grey pallor, which others can see some twenty to thirty minutes before the patient complains of feeling ill. The brain function is disturbed; memory, concentration, and emotional ups and downs are usual. Patients can fail to understand what they read, be unable to judge distances, have sweating and dizziness on standing, and have sleep alteration with vivid dreams. In every case the symptoms fluctuate in severity throughout the course of a day. Most cases make a recovery within a few years, but the disease has an alarming tendency to become chronic in about a quarter of all cases.

Dr Ramsay, the key doctor involved in the London hospital epidemic, with a distinguished record in the area of infectious diseases, had worked in Africa before being appointed to a consultant's post at the Royal Free Hospital. He was not the only British doctor to witness and report on an epidemic of ME. Nine years later, in 1964, three hundred and seventy cases of ME occurred, mainly in the practice of Dr Betty Scott in Finchley. Dr Scott reported her findings to the BMJ in 1970. In 1970 and 1971, one hundred and forty-five cases, mainly hospital workers, were affected by an outbreak at Great Ormond Street Hospital for Sick Children. Some cases of ill children were referred to the hospital with symptoms but no records were kept.

For many years the name Myalgic Encephalomyelitis (ME) was accepted, as was the illness, and by 1986 – when he wrote his second book about the disease – Dr Ramsay had discovered that the illness was a world-wide phenomenon. All the outbreaks had similar symptoms but had been given different names. The name Myalgic Encephalomyelitis was put forward in 1978 by a leader writer in the BMJ, but Royal Free disease, Epidemic Neuromyesthenia, Icelandic disease and Atypical Poliomyelitis were also used.

By 1986 Dr Ramsay had identified outbreaks ranging from Switzerland to Australia, Washington and Iceland and from South Africa to Florida as well as discovering other outbreaks in different parts of Britain. Following on from the Royal Free in 1955, a Dr John Richardson had reported cases in Cumbria, and subsequently cases appeared in Newcastle and Great Ormond Street Hospital for Sick Children in London. By 1984 not only was a Dr Bell in New York dealing with 200 cases, of whom 35 were adolescents and children, but there was an epidemic at Lake Tahoe, USA, which had started with a girls' basketball team and went on to infect three High Schools and then spread to the community. The physical nature of the disease, as Dr Ramsay confidently observed, was becoming self evident.

The earliest report that Dr Ramsay uncovered was from Los Angeles in 1934, where at first the epidemic was considered to be poliomyelitis. (Poliomyelitis is a viral disease that can affect nerves and can lead to partial or full paralysis). Several subsequent epidemics occurred where poliomyelitis had been present. In Iceland in 1948-1949 there had been an epidemic of poliomyelitis. However, in regions where epidemic neuromyasthenia had occurred, poliomyelitis did not spread. In Adelaide, Australia in 1949-1950 poliomyelitis had been spreading at an alarming rate yet, almost overnight, the cases of poliomyelitis stopped and seven hundred reported cases of ME replaced them. (The difference was confirmed by the samples of cerebrospinal fluid; there was evidence of the usual changes in the cerebrospinal fluid in the poliomyelitis cases but none in the ME cases). Significantly, in Britain in the early 1950s, a widespread epidemic of poliomyelitis had been raging.

Before the Royal Free outbreak Dr E. D. Acheson had described an outbreak of an infectious disease involving the nervous system and the muscles among fourteen nurses at the Middlesex hospital in 1952.

In 1953 in Coventry an outbreak resembling poliomyelitis had broken out where some of the nurses working on the polio wards experienced upper respiratory symptoms, lethargy, nausea, chills, general muscle weakness and concentration difficulties, lasting for two months or more. Their tests were clear but they did show antibodies against poliomyelitis and therefore this was not the reason for their illness.

At a teachers' training college in Newcastle in 1959 out of one hundred and twenty students, fifty became ill. What was remarkable about this epidemic is that only two of the nuns who shared the college building became ill. In Los Angeles the largest outbreak involved one hundred and ninety-eight members of the medical and nursing staff.

In the 1955 Royal Free epidemic two hundred and ninety-two members of the medical and nursing staff were affected but only twelve patients became ill although the hospital was full at the time. Prior to the Royal Free epidemic, in February of that year, there had been a similar outbreak in Durban in South Africa amongst ninety-eight nurses. The pattern that became apparent from these and other epidemics was of active people becoming ill while the more sedentary escaped.

From the very first epidemic in Britain the doctors involved have carried out blood, muscle and neurological tests. Unfortunately, in sporadic cases the patient presents too late for tests to show any active agent. Dr Ramsay and his colleagues said that their results showed a pattern closely similar to Duchenne Muscular Dystrophy, the hereditary muscle wasting disease. Dr Betty Scott noticed hypoglycaemia which is low blood sugar level, unusual nerve tests and facial pallor. The laboratory investigation findings from the Great Ormond Street outbreak were in abnormalities in the immune system.

The Scottish cases in West Kilbride in Ayrshire, Balfron in Stirlingshire and Helensburgh in Argyll and Bute in the 1980s were all studied and compared with healthy adults. Professor P. Behan was able to show changes in illnesses that he grouped under 'Post infectious encephalomyelitis.' These changes included unusual white blood cell presentations in the blood, abnormal findings in the spinal fluid and changes in muscle testing with electromyography. He also found that the patients had raised antibodies against the coxsackie B virus. Their main observation, exemplified in one case where two members of one family, a father and his eight-year-old daughter both had the illness, was that one of the triggering factors for a person to contract the illness was the state of the individual's immune system at the time.

By the end of 1999 Dr John Richardson, who had been the doctor involved with the cases in Cumbria which occurred at the same time as the Royal Free epidemic, had followed up cases for forty years. He compiled a comprehensive list of abnormal findings; to help other doctors to spot the illness he devised a check list of symptoms. He also raised some alarm bells about what happened to the babies of ME patients. Dr Richardson found that if a mother's serum tests were positive to enteroviruses then there was a likelihood of the baby being born with a central nervous system defect. Enteroviruses enter the body via the gastrointestinal tract and thrive there, often moving on to attack the nervous system. Polioviruses and coxsackie viruses are enteroviruses. Dr Richardson found that where he had treated the mothers with IgG – an immunoglobulin which can pass through the placenta – the babies were normal. It was apparent to all these doctors that they were dealing with an organic or physical disease.

However, in early 1970s two psychiatrists had queried the findings. They had been given permission to examine the records of the Royal Free outbreak and the result was that one of the doctors, a Mr McEvedy, decided to do a PhD proposing that the illnesses were, in reality, manifestations of mass hysteria. This was lapped up by the media. Although the medical council urged caution, the diagnosis rocked the profession and the possibility of ME having a psychiatric cause began to infiltrate the profession.

The doubts around the physical nature of Myalgic Encephalitis persisted. In 1986 a young boy in the Isle of Man, Ean Proctor, was diagnosed with severe ME. On his second visit to his consultant in London a psychiatrist named Simon Wessely took an interest in his case. Dr Wessely, along with others in Britain and America, was sceptical about unevidenced illnesses such as ME, and he suggested that the boy might help with their research.

Dr Wessely's report stated that Ean's apparent illness was 'out of all proportion to the original cause' and 'I feel that Ean needs a long period of rehabilitation, part of which will involve very skilled management of separation from his parents'.

Across the Atlantic similar beliefs were expounded at the inquiry into the Lake Tahoe outbreak. It was at this symposium, in 1986, that the term Chronic Fatigue Syndrome (CFS) was coined, and from that moment ME became subsumed into this umbrella term and called CFS/ME. Management for the condition became one of a psychiatric approach to change a patient's false illness beliefs, with graded exercise.

ME was unlucky in the timing of its arrival on the medical scene and the manner in which it presented itself. Rarely is ME fatal, although those suffering it are likely to die at an earlier age than their healthier counterparts. ME, in sporadic cases, is not dramatic. Nothing is seen once the person has got over the original illness, and this first illness is short lived. It does not leave the person paralysed, nor does it leave any traces of disease in any tests. These factors place it low in the order of priority when it comes to mobilising research. ME arrived at a time when medicine was moving towards surgical interventions which substantially changed people's lives. New joints were enabling people to walk again. Organ replacement and repair were restoring otherwise dying people to a full life. Cancer and heart conditions were beginning to be more successfully detected and treated.

ME was listed by the World Health Organisation (WHO) as a disease of the nervous system. Neurological illnesses were having to take a back seat. ME makes only a small burden on the health service. Those who suffer from it soon disappear from surgeries. They also disappear from schools, workplaces and society. ME patients becomes hidden. ME has done this so successfully that its very existence is questioned.

It was in 1986 as this controversy was brewing, and in an area of Ayrshire, Scotland, where twenty-two patients who were suspected of having contracted ME between 1980 and 1983 were being investigated, that Chris, our son, was born.

1996-2001

Time hovers o'er, impatient to destroy
And shuts up all the passages of joy.

Samuel Johnson

Myalgic Encephalomyelitis is a difficult illness to describe, in that so many of those suffering from it look no different from those that are healthy. It is in their capabilities that they are deficient, their lack of energy, their extreme fatigue following exercise, which is often manifest several days later, and the feeling that they have that their bodies are poisoned. That is the essence of ME. Degrees of the condition vary, as is the case with most neurological diseases, and it can vary from mild, where the person suffers symptoms after playing sport or working for exams, to severe where even reading or speaking is impossible. These patients do not exhibit any abnormalities in any routine medical tests. This is the crux of the controversy. How can people be so ill, and yet show a blank on testing? People can live with the condition for months or years and there is no indication of why they are not functioning normally. It is for this reason that the question can be asked, is this not a psychiatric disorder?

In 1996 no one in our family had any knowledge of ME; it was not until Chris was about nine years old that he began to show signs of becoming regularly unwell. The first incidence of any significance connected with his health was when Chris ran into the kitchen, more upset than usual. He had been playing football with his eldest brother Iain and the ball had hit the back of his head. Nothing would persuade him to return outside.

By the next day he was unable to move his neck in any direction. When it did not ease up I took him to our doctor, who referred him to a consultant. Although I am a physiotherapist and had examined him, I could find no obvious reason for his immobility. At school, they adapted his desk so that he could write on a slant; by the end of the term he was almost back to normal. Except, that is, for his maths and his music.

Chris, aged ten, was going to a new school in the autumn. We had been doing some extra maths so that he would be more confident when settling into his new class. He actually enjoyed it; we would go through the book at odd moments such as when waiting to pick up his older brother, Dougal, from his cricket fixtures. Suddenly he was making mistakes everywhere. It was illogical to believe that he was unable to do the work because of the neck injury, yet there was no other explanation.

At the same time Chris had been preparing for Grade 1 on the piano. Inexplicably he was making mistakes where previously he had not. His teacher could only presume that he had got cold feet and recommended that he restart lessons once he was at his new school.

It is difficult to know what Chris thought at that time; he was naturally ready for a challenge and there must have been a sense of unease that his body had become temporarily unpredictable. What other explanation could there be than that his hand-eye-maths-music connections had been affected by the injury? When we saw the consultant two months later all symptoms had receded, and he could find nothing amiss, and he looked rather quizzically at me when I mention the music and the maths.

The first year at his new school was exhilarating and challenging. Chris, his cousin Helen, and another slightly older boy, James, travelled by train to and from the school. He made new friends, started new sports and enjoyed the new routine that a larger school could offer.

The nights, however, were a different matter. Night after night Chris would end up sleeping on a mattress at the foot of our bed. He would rarely be asleep before we went upstairs.

Sometimes I would wake to find a shadowy figure standing by my bed. At other times I would hear a noise on the landing between our rooms and would find Chris standing under the light that we always left on, frozen with fear. We presumed that this was a legacy from the burglary.

The burglary had occurred a year before. We lived in a remote farmhouse on the edge of a village on the west coast of Scotland. One night in July 1996 two men entered the house. Dougal, aged eighteen, was watching television. Chris, my husband Alex and I were asleep upstairs. Iain, aged nineteen, was away at the time. Dougal was assaulted from behind and thereafter taken at knife point around the house as the men stole at random. It was once they found the cartridges that they became very excited, and insisted that Dougal take them to our room so as to gain access to our guns. At some point during the nightmare they asked Dougal who slept in the other bedroom. He answered that it belonged to his wee brother and they decided to leave him alone. Although Chris slept through the ordeal he wrote his version of the burglary five years later.

Chris' story

'Excuse me, could you tell me the time, please?' My whole family jumped at this innocuous question, something we would never have done before the previous evening's drama.

As we headed for the police station to have our finger prints taken, I realised that I would never feel the same about a stranger again.

Usually when asked a question like this I would react as if it was one of my friends or family asking me a question, but this was different. By nature I was a generally trusting person, but the circumstances had changed me. I was suspicious of everybody.

The circumstance was a burglary. The suspicion that anybody could do anything to you at any time. The day before the day in question was the day that had changed my life. At 9.00pm a man had come to our door to ask if he could hire a fishing pass. 'Strange' we thought, as it was getting on and by the time he had reached the river it would be very late. But we let it go. We filtered off to bed one at a time and eventually only my brother Dougal was left downstairs. He heard the door open. From then on he was traipsed round the house for two hours. My Mum and Dad were tied up as I slept through banging doors, shouting and screams - maybe there is a God! I was woken by my Mum and we promptly set off for the local pub, where we spent most of the night.

So this brings me to the present day where I am still feeling the effects of this 'adventure' as my oldest brother described it. He was on holiday at the time.

In some ways the burglary was an interesting experience. This may seem insane to someone who has ever had to go through the whole ordeal of working out what has been taken, courtroom battles, and fingerprinting, but it really opens your eyes to the outside world. It took me a few days to realise, but when I did it totally changed my life. It made me realise how incredibly naïve I had been for the nine previous years of my life. I, along with my family, had always watched the evening news about recent burglaries or murders and thought 'It will never happen to me'. How wrong! Not only did it bring me crashing *down to earth, but it pinned my eyes and especially my ears wide open. So wide at night that, between the same hours as the two men entered our house and burgled it, I can still, at the age of fourteen, hardly ever sleep. Slowly it is becoming easier but I still sit bolt upright, as if I had a spring in my body, if I hear a louder than average creak in the house.*

The other interesting thing about the burglary was the way possessions suddenly seemed worthless when your families' lives are at risk. I didn't mind if my beloved stereo was packed into a car and driven off never to be seen again. The only thing I could think about were the 'what if's'. What if my brother had made a mistake, or said something wrong as he was traipsed round the house at knifepoint? My mind churns over the options. But something I can say for sure is that I hope I shall never experience that kind of fear again.

As a result of the burglary Chris began to sleep poorly and I would be aware, since I too suffered from disturbed nights, that Chris was standing on the landing outside our room too scared to move. On other occasions he would be unable to sleep until we went upstairs, and then we would put him on a mattress at the foot of our bed. Many children dislike sleeping alone so, when neither of his brothers were around to share his room, or he did not have friends to stay, I would move into the other bed in his room. I was to sleep there, whenever it was necessary, for the next three years. Alex and I thought it was a small price to pay for peace of mind, never thinking that this situation would persist so long.

About a year later, three weeks before we were due to leave for Iain's wedding in USA, Chris became ill. After a fortnight of lying listlessly on the sofa, unable to do work sent from school, feeling hot but with a low temperature, pale and uninterested in food, he took a turn for the worse. I began to wonder if someone was going to have to stay behind to look after him. His temperature was raging. "Mum, can you just hold me?" he asked. I rang the evening duty doctor who thought it unlikely that he had meningitis but was unable to advise us. Miraculously, a few days later he was well enough to travel.

The summer was a cricketing dream for Chris, who not only captained his school team but also played regularly at the local club. When the autumn term started, his enthusiastic sports master asked him if he could play rugby. I had consistently refused him permission the year before because of his recurrent neck problem. "Can't you ask your Mother to treat it for you?" We had a few sessions but his was not like other necks that I treated. Usually a person with a sore neck will present with some of the joints tender and stiff, but the joints on both sides of Chris' were acutely tender and he had no apparent joint stiffness at all.

Odd incidents would force Chris to have a week off school, an exceptionally cold rugby session, an anaesthetic to remove a tooth, a weekend staying away with school friends, a school trip to France. "I never see any reason to send my children on school trips," was the unhelpful comment I received, from one of our GPs, when I tried to explain how these events would trigger his illness.

I would dread the telltale signs heralding another spell off school. The forty minutes that Chris would spend on his roller blades when he got home from school would reduce to thirty, then twenty, then ten over consecutive days and then he would not go out at all. Sometimes he would say 'this yoghurt is off' when it was not. Iain would tell Chris to go and clean his teeth because his breath smelt so unpleasant. Or Iain would say in exasperation, "Mum, would you please feed him!" because he noticed that Chris was less irritable after his supper. He appeared to have less stamina than the other boys of his age.

On one occasion when I took him to the doctor he asked Chris, "What do you think is the matter with you?" "I can't sleep," he replied. I noticed when he was asleep that he was never still and made small movements all the time. He would come down to breakfast heavy-lidded and white-faced, force down cereal and sausages but become more lively as we travelled to the bus. Some days he would appear almost drugged and, although all dressed for school, say, "I just can't go today." This would lead to another few days on the sofa. The pattern of illness was always the same. I tried keeping food diaries and noted the dates that he was off school. It seemed that in winter he would be ill for one week in every five. He would be pale, listless, disinterested and disinclined to eat. He just stayed in the TV room and life continued around him. I felt almost guilty that he required so little attention. He barely wanted to play cards or board games or raise an interest in all the things that he usually enjoyed doing. I would carry on with all my activities. His recovery was always as if a switch had been turned on. Each time you were able to believe that it would not happen again.

One incident occurred during those three years at that school which I remembered with misgivings at a much later date. The train from school had been delayed. It was a warm afternoon, so it was no hardship to wander up and down the platform or sit on a low wall in the sun. It was a small station and only one or two other people were waiting. I recognised another parent and we started talking. I was absorbed as I listened to the father's story about his daughter. Any medical condition intrigues me and here was a girl, at the top of her field as a junior equestrian, who became so ill that even although she was recovering she was still only attending school part-time. She had had three successive bouts of tonsillitis and had subsequently missed school for a year. When I related this story to another mother she remarked unsympathetically, "Those parents always pushed that child."

The school accepted Chris' absences and he managed to keep up with the work, although he no longer challenged himself against the brighter children as he used to, and he gave up playing chess.

"I find some children don't cope very well once they move up to secondary," the deputy head said to me during one parents' evening. I believed that Chris was managing better than expected, considering the amount of school he had missed. Since joining the school Chris had been thoroughly content; it was his health that was the problem.

"Perhaps he has ME." Alex said, exasperated, after Chris had yet another spell of illness. I was shocked. ME was not like this. You were ill for months, not just the odd week; what did he know about it, anyway? Almost immediately I dismissed the idea; it was too terrible a diagnosis to contemplate; it was inconceivable. Chris' symptoms did not resemble those described by a colleague. I could barely pronounce myalgic encephalomyelitis, let alone grasp the concept. I did not think it had any relevance to Chris' school absences and never gave it another thought.

I did wonder about a diagnosis of something sinister such as leukaemia but then I ruled this out because the erratic nature of his symptoms were incompatible with the inexorable march of cancer. Cancer would show on a blood test I reasoned. On another visit to the doctor he reported that all the tests were clear. They could find nothing wrong with him. "But he is still ill." I said. "Oh! I can see he's ill," he responded, and referred Chris to a consultant paediatrician. I was convinced an easy answer would be found. It was now four years since the burglary and three years since this pattern of illness had started. We needed answers!

"Chris is ill roughly every five weeks," I began at our consultation with the paediatrician. "When he is unwell it lasts about a week. He is pale and he cannot do anything. He seems to be hot, but his temperature is sometimes even below normal. Paracetomol does not help; in fact it seems to make him worse. Extra activities such as a school trip will trigger things." This was all I could think to tell him.

Outside, the waiting room was full and I felt the constraints on the consultant's time. The room was small, the ceilings low, the walls covered in cheery posters and children's pictures. Low tables, toys and children filled the floor space. How could I mention my misgivings about his stamina, his music and his maths? I felt as if I were making excuses for an underachieving child. To a doctor it would certainly be interpreted as such. He would not want to hear about Chris' neck; we had had that checked out. The reaction to food could be explained away with the thought, probably unspoken, of 'fussy eater'. I could detect that he had lost his edge in cricket and only I knew that if I did not oversee and encourage all his piano and 'cello practices he would give up. I knew he needed me to prompt or guide him. I had to do the same with his homework. Anyone observing could describe me as an overprotective mother, but he just could not function without my input. It would be so easy to give a quasi-psychological explanation but I knew that fundamentally something was wrong.

The consultant looked at all his previous tests, which were negative, and took new samples of blood for a battery of further tests. He gave Chris a very careful and attentive examination, despite the irritation of phone calls and the need to include a student who was shadowing. He reassured us. "I really can find nothing to be alarmed about," he said, "I think you will find that when you have moved and started afresh in Edinburgh, there will be a significant improvement."

It was true. Radical changes had taken place in our lives. My husband, Alex, had stood for and gained a place in the new Scottish Parliament. He had been selected to represent Galloway and Upper Nithsdale. Our lives would now be split between Kirkcudbrightshire and Edinburgh. There would be no more travelling as Chris' new school would be just a ten minute walk away from our Edinburgh flat.

The Under 15 cricket team had club fixtures every Friday. There was one last cricket fixture that summer before we left Ayrshire. Colin was one of two twenty-year-old players from the 1st Eleven who accompanied and cheerfully supervised the team to their matches. Towards the end of the game I had a chance to thank Colin and his friend. I also had a chance to ask them about their lives and line of work. "I'm going to Australia for a year," said Colin, "to play cricket and travel." My face must have shown some surprise as they were obviously no longer students. "He should have gone to Australia with me," his friend explained, "but Colin was ill for three years and missed out on University."

"I had something called ME," said Colin.

On our first evening in Edinburgh, Chris came in waving a £20 note. He had been looking out of his bedroom window, watching, bemused, the unfamiliar urban scene. We had moved into a ground floor flat that day. It was in the centre of town and we had neighbours, and locked doors, and people walking by on the pavement. Chris had spotted the note being blown along tossed by the wind. The pavements *were* made of gold. Perhaps this was an omen.

"Mum, I've never been so scared in all my life. For the first hour I was just shaking all the time," Chris said at the end of his first day at school. He was exhilarated, however, and by the third day had walked home with a friend. Chris' initiation had been slightly more daunting than I had envisaged. There were two hundred boys in the second year and only four of them were new. It takes a while before firm friendships are made, sports teams joined, and a social life emerges. For the first few weeks life was uneventful.

The flat was conveniently on the route between the school and the station, so Chris started inviting friends in when they were heading home. At other times he would accompany them up to the town. He was man of the match in an inter-house football tournament. Encouraged by a friend he went to the second-year disco night. When the winter nets started he joined in anticipation for the eagerly awaited cricket season. I felt that life was returning to normal.

I had to go and look after my Mother for a week during the spring term. Since the school had boarding facilities I arranged for Chris to stay there. His initial reluctance was soon dispelled when he encountered the joys of evenings playing table tennis or snooker or football. Unfortunately, cricket, coupled with the week in the boarding house, where it was too much fun to go to bed, provoked a return of his illness.

On the Sunday afternoon before I was due back Chris had a training session with the East of Scotland Under15 cricket team at Cramond. The house tutor volunteered to deliver and collect him. The session finished at 5.30, when it was already dark. Chris walked through the old Training School grounds to the gate as arranged and waited. A few of the other people who were leaving gave him a wave; his coach stopped to ask if he was being collected before he drove home. Chris waited for an hour at the edge of the dark, tree-lined and relatively little-used road. He became unable to move as his fears grew, and if he had been able to, where would he go? He told me later that his mind became full of terrifying scenarios as he became more and more frightened. Finally he made himself retrace his route back to the hall. The car park was dimly lit but for the last hundred yards the path led between two unlit buildings. Fortunately the Under19s were still training. The tutor apologised when I collected Chris two days later and I made light of it, as did Chris. I was not surprised when Chris' old symptoms returned but inwardly I was beginning to feel scared. Nothing had changed; Chris was not going to have a trouble-free secondary schooling.

Chris decided to invite some friends to stay with us in Cornwall that summer. Along with two of his new school friends he naturally thought to invite Helen, whose Mother had recently died. There was plenty to do, with volley ball and table tennis in the garden, and a beach only eight hundred yards from the house. Two days before the end of the holiday, the morning after they had all had a long surf on a particularly cold day, Chris arrived to breakfast ahead of the others, stating that he felt unwell. I said that I would entertain his friends; he spent the last two days resting his head on his arms at the kitchen table, watching the Test Match. There was the thought that Chris' nose might be out of joint because of the extra attention that I was giving to Helen. I had spent a small part of each day helping to dry her hair, hoping that this contact might fill part of the gap left by her Mother's death. Chris rallied a bit by the time we were on our way home.

A few days after our return there was the last cricket match of the season. His club were playing against another team, several of whose members were in the District Squad. Chris had forgotten about the fixture until an hour before the match was due, which in itself was, in retrospect, out of character. I managed to drop him off at the ground just in time. Later I went to watch some of the game. I can remember looking at the scoreboard when I arrived and seeing a healthy forty runs against his position. He looked confident and elated when the match was over. This was much more like his old form and would bode well for the next season. At least the year had ended on a buoyant note. Little did we know that this would be his swan-song.

A week later Chris pulled up sharply in P.E. His neck was extremely painful and would not move. Alex took him to be checked at the hospital but nothing was injured. We cancelled a trip to London for a family and friends cricket match. A week's rest enabled Chris to recover. Now that he was in third year there were more opportunities available to him. There was Army cadet corps and Duke of Edinburgh, football and friends to stay. We had also arranged to have a holiday in the October fortnight, visiting Iain and Becca in North Carolina.

When we were in North Carolina, Iain had organised three nights in the Smokey Blue Mountains, staying in a wooden chalet in Bear Wallow. We enjoyed clambering through the forest surrounding the chalet. One day we went boating and swimming in the chilly lake. Another day we went white-water rafting, which was also rather a chilly experience. On the final day we decided to follow a trail to the Grey Mare's Tail. We climbed through the thick evergreen forest. As we did so, the pine trees slowly thinned to give way to tall deciduous trees. Encouraged by those people coming down who told us the effort was worth it, we continued upwards until the sun began to filter through. The trees diminished in size and the colours of the leaves increased in variety and intensity. Finally we emerged, not at a waterfall as we had anticipated but at a huge flat overhanging rock. It was like a roof from which we could see, in the brilliant sunlight and as far as the horizon, acres and acres of red, yellow, and orange trees covering every peak of every mountainside. This was the Fall that we had heard about. The descent took only an hour. Iain and Chris would disappear ahead of us, and Becca and I would discover them sitting on a rock in a Buddha pose, or surprising us from behind. This was a holiday we would have reason to remember, because it would be a very long time before he had another.

On the return journey Chris' right leg went into a spasm and would not straighten. I recalled an occasion when walking with him in Edinburgh over a year before that his leg had behaved in a similar fashion and his knee would not stretch. Odd things did happen to him.

Once, when I had gone to say goodnight to him, he said, "It was really strange, Mum, when I was going up the stairs my left arm went out to the side all by itself."

I made light of it at the time and soon forgot the incident.

The following morning Chris was covered in a rash. It was warm but not really warm enough for prickly heat. Two days after we arrived home in Scotland, the rash re-appeared.

Soon after this the Army corps had a weekend exercise. Armed with water bottle, plastic plate, mug and all the other paraphernalia, Chris joined his troop. Under their charismatic leader they spent two days stalking other troops, lying in wait in bogs, and finally meeting up for the gruelling stretcher run. It seems that Chris excelled himself in this task which involved running in relays with a 'body', as I understood it. Exhausting anyway.

At the time we did not link the Army exercise with Chris' next bout of illness and absence from school. Following it, Chris managed to go intermittently to school but everything was now an effort. On Tuesdays I worked late and would leave Chris to make his own supper, but when Alex arrived home he would discover that Chris still had not eaten. Once again Maths was proving difficult and doing any homework required encouragement. I would wake and find him at 1 am busily doing the homework with which he had struggled earlier. He no longer relished jaunts to Princes Street with his friends and that upset him, as he wondered what was happening to him. I had noticed in the summer that I had to alter my pace when walking with him and had to slow down. How could a fourteen-year-old have less energy than his mother? He was doing less than he had for ages. There was no travelling to school or extras such as music. He was not playing rugby and recently he had begun to miss the Army corps and the Duke of Edinburgh evenings. Yet he was feeling faint in Assembly and fell unaccountably on the way to school. He had to force down breakfast and take lucozade tablets with him each day to try and keep going. Then came the day when, unable even to play his Play Station game of Championship Manager, which had become his chief preoccupation at weekends, Chris lay in front of the television with his feet up on a stool under a duvet. He felt wretched, answered any questions with short economical answers, and I was sufficiently alarmed to make an appointment with the doctor. Our GP was patient, listened carefully and took some blood samples but the tests returned clear. Chris had missed, I calculated, almost as many days as he had attended at school that term. By the end of November he was back in school again. But not for long.

Christmas with our relations was very lazy and partly due to a sore foot Chris had a good rest. Several inches of snow had fallen while we were away. On our return home we had to abandon the car and stomp through the snow for the final eight hundred yards up the track to our house. The next morning we woke to a stunning sunlit snowy scene. Alex took Chris to the surgery for a follow-up blood test and then he and I took out the sledges. The steep hill beside the house made an excellent sledge track although the bend proved trickier than anticipated. I trudged back up after our first run, to join Chris at the top. As I rounded the corner I saw him lying spread-eagled on the snow. "What's up?" I asked and something in his voice sent a chill through me. He replied "I can't get up."

This time Chris really was ill. He was pale, monosyllabic, sweating, too hot, too cold, unable to concentrate and unable to sleep. Twice he came through to see me in the night to say that his heart was 'thumping so hard and so fast'. I was now very anxious. We returned to the GP and

I wrote out everything that I could remember to try and help him with a diagnosis.

"You know, there are many occasions when doctors simply do not know what causes a person to be ill. We can probably only make a diagnosis in twenty-five per cent of the cases that come to our surgery," the doctor told me, but he arranged for ultrasound tests on his kidneys. The results from these tests were clear.

The GP referred us to our former Paediatrician. We were very much more apprehensive as we left for this second visit to the Consultant. Chris was more noticeably ill this time as compared to our previous consultation eighteen months before. Both Alex and I accompanied him.

I knew the hospital well, as I had worked there for five years. From the warm safety of being a member of staff I was here like any other child's mother, scared and on unfamiliar territory. Time and again I had scoured the medical books to try and analyse what could be wrong with Chris but nothing made sense. I just knew this recurrent illness could not be common because none of his school friends or his brothers' school friends or anyone I knew had anything similar to this.

I suspect that the Consultant had slotted us into his timetable, especially since we were seeing him on the ward and not at his clinic, and I appreciated his efforts on our behalf. I feared that the examination again might not give us an answer. I was not prepared, however, for his eventual recommendation.

Chris lay on the bed, eerily still for a boy of his age, replying economically to any questions and without any extraneous movements. This stillness was usual when he was feeling ill. The Consultant did a thorough examination and he was kind and gentle.

"I will send off for a muscle enzyme test but I don't really expect to find anything abnormal." The Consultant said as he drew the interview to a close and gave a despairing shrug. "My only suggestion is, that you consult a psychiatrist."

As we walked back along the corridors towards the canteen I felt so relieved that Alex had come with me to this interview. How could I have explained to him that the examination had elicited no diagnosis and that Chris could have a mental health problem? Alex and I were in agreement when we discussed this over coffee in the hospital canteen. No-one would ever put their child in the hands of a psychiatrist when the main therapy at their disposal is drug therapy.

We were aware that Chris, like ourselves, had found the burglary shocking in its emotional and psychological impact, but nothing had ever led us to believe that Chris had a mental illness. Chris joined us with his drink and sat down.

"What did he say we should do, that you say that we are not going to do?" Chris asked.

"Go to a psychiatrist." Alex answered.

"Why would he suggest that?"

"Because he can't find anything the matter with you."

There was a pause as Chris looked down at his drink.

"That means," he said, with more energy than we had seen for a while, "that he thinks that it's all in my head. That means that he does not believe me."

2001 Spring

"The best way to fill time is to waste it"

Marguerite Duras

During the first year of Chris' illness many of my previously held assumptions about medicine were challenged. Until 1996, when Chris started having mysterious spells of illness, medicine was simple. There was a pathology for each illness, and once a diagnosis was established, a treatment and a prognosis would be given. The pathology told you what was happening to the body and why it was not functioning correctly, and the prognosis gave you an idea of the course that the illness would take, including when you might expect to be better.

Combined with this is a respect for doctors, for their knowledge and their position in society. The doctor is the gateway to accessing health services. He is the guardian of our health. Recently patients have been encouraged to take a more active role in the treatment and rehabilitation of their health problems, yet the very fact that in Britain we have a free service mitigates against the patient. The patient has essentially a passive part to play because he does not pay. If the funding followed the patient there would be more options open, as in the USA, because he would be in the driving seat. If a doctor has no answer to a problem the patient is left powerless to seek further within the system.

Chris was given no diagnosis, therefore there was no treatment, no plan, nor acknowledgement that he was ill. He was suddenly on the outside of established conventional medicine. I was to have to take the position as physician and carer. As a physiotherapist I had had a conventional medical training, yet now I was on my own. I would be the focus of attention as I struggled to make the decisions necessary to manage my child's illness. With no other guidance than instinct and what reading matter I could lay my hands on, I embarked into unknown territory. Quickly carers become socially isolated. They are 'damned if they do and damned if they don't'. If they stay at home they are condemned for being over-protective. Neglectful if they go to work. They make decisions for their child in the absence of a doctor's endorsement, yet many doctors' guidelines can be seen as misguided and detrimental to their child's recovery. The opprobrium that can be heaped on the mother by the establishment is then, reasonably, copied by society. The child and the mother can be, and are, ignored by both.

At the beginning of 2001 Chris went to school on the second day of term, but that was the last day that he attended. With no diagnosis, but increasingly unwell, I wondered what to do.

What is this illness? An answer arrived sooner than we expected. Alex had received an e-mail from Helen McDade, who has a child with ME and is on the Edinburgh self-help group.

"What about a Cross-Party group for ME?" She wrote to all the MSPs.

"Why do we need one?" Alex replied.

"That's why." Helen replied enigmatically. Alex was intrigued enough to go to their inaugural meeting.

When Alex came home after the meeting he told me that while listening to the speakers he felt certain that Chris was suffering from ME. He had stayed behind to speak to the two doctors, both of whom are sufferers of ME who work as and when their ME permits them. One of them, Dr Mason Brown, runs a clinic near Edinburgh; he gave him some helpful hand-outs and a tape. The other was Dr Vance Spence from Dundee, who is a researcher into vascular (blood) disorders.

He advised Alex to see a Dr Speight, a paediatric consultant working in Durham with great experience of children with ME. He advised us not to seek a referral to any Edinburgh consultant because we would in all probability be referred to a psychiatrist. It would be possible to arrange a consultation through our GP in Galloway. The word spread around our family and friends that we had a possible diagnosis for Chris and through the post we were sent sheaves of information downloaded from the Internet. The more I read the more the symptoms corresponded with those we had observed over the years. I was even able to find explanations for symptoms which I had not known were connected.

MYALGIC = pain in the muscles
ENCEPHALO = brain function involvement
MYELITIS = inflammation of the nerve sheaths

The most common symptoms are fatigue, both mental and physical, malaise or feeling poisoned, persistent headache, disturbed sleep, brain disturbance.

Eye pain or blurring, sensitivity to light and sound, altered temperature control, balance disturbance on change of position especially from lying to standing, recurrent sore throat, nausea or feeling sick, loss of appetite, muscle or joint pains, mood changes out of character, and facial pallor. Symptoms can fluctuate, but key symptoms are common to all patients: fatigue after minimal effort, malaise [feeling very ill], and cognitive [thinking] dysfunction are invariably present. The disease tends to relapse and have remissions over months.

*Myalgic Encephalomyelitis is an **endemic** disease that has **epidemic** outbreaks. This presentation of the disease is the most common but it is not taught to medical students. The number of doctors or their wives who suffer is quite out of proportion to their numbers in the population as a whole. The main features of the disease come under three headings. 1/ muscle phenomena whereby even after minor degrees of physical effort three to five days elapse before full muscle power is restored. 2/ circulatory impairment with hypersensitivity to temperature change and the observable ashen-grey facial pallor. 3/ cerebral dysfunction or brain fog. The final property of ME is that although most cases make a complete recovery over a few years, it has an alarming tendency to become chronic and at a conservative estimate the figure is 25%. In these cases the disease lasts for years and years, in some the disease relapses and goes into remission, in the others no remission occurs.*

I knew that I would understand about ME and believe in it if I could hear about it at first hand.

The son of the present Headmaster of the primary school that I used to attend had had ME. I remember being told that their boy had been so ill that his parents had to turn him at night. Our telephone conversation lasted nearly an hour and as the headmaster's story of his son's six year illness unfolded I realised that here was a disease that followed no recognisable pattern. Far from encountering sympathy and compassion, the family had been subjected to disbelief and ridicule. The boy, aged twelve, fell ill after a rugby festival lasting two days and following his BCG injection. He became progressively more ill but was accused of trying to avoid school and of being school-phobic. As he got weaker he was admitted to hospital where he was subjected to tilt table tests and, only after being thrown into a swimming pool, convinced the medical profession that he was so weak he could not swim. "I can still remember the look in his eyes," his father said as he recalled watching his son being subjected to this ordeal. While he was talking I could imagine the sense of betrayal that the father must have felt towards his son, and the utter loss of control that patients feel in the face of the medical profession. "Eventually we decided to remove him from the hospital and undertook to care for him ourselves."

He explained how unpopular a disease ME is. Also that a diagnosis of ME can be an invitation to social services and the medical profession to enforce their views (that ME is a somatic illness - an illness of the mind manifested in the body) on a very sick child.

The headmaster went on to give me advice on healthy eating, avoiding quack remedies, and outlined his son's slow rehabilitation. All this time I had a feeling of unreality, surely this was a worst case scenario, this would not happen to us. He gave me two pieces of advice. "Don't give up your work." His wife had employed a carer to help during the day and she continued with her job, while they both covered the nights. They rigged up a line from their room to their son's so that he could call them, though he admitted that he used to dread the sound of the bell. Secondly, something else that his wife had done, "Keep a diary."

I found a 2000 diary from the Republic of China, I had no idea how we had acquired it but it was hard-backed, a reasonable size and being from the previous year I could write anywhere and disregard the dates. I turned to the very last double page spread; this covered December 25-31 and was divided into six days - Saturday and Sunday shared a section.

Two lines up from the bottom of the page I started a graph heading towards the front of the diary. I wrote 'Dec 29th - sledging' against it. The first line went across the page, mainly slipping downwards and I marked 'Jan 10th, Feb 1st, Feb 14th' and then started across the adjacent page. Underneath the graph I wrote. 'In bed. Bath every 3-4 days. Sleep mostly poor. Skin sweating'.

I had started a diary of ME.

February 14th

We had an invitation from the parents of Dougal's girlfriend Katie to go to a UNICEF charity dance that they have organised. As it is two hours from Edinburgh they invited us to stay the night. Chris is not well enough to be left overnight but Alex insisted that we accept. "He can rest on their sofa just as well as on ours. We have to continue with some semblance of normal life." Katie's parents were happy for us to take him with us.

When we arrived at their cottage we were unable to park by the door but had to climb up some thirty steps. Normally this would have been unremarkable but I am beginning to realize that any extra exertion leaves Chris feeling worse. It is ridiculous that a flight of steps could challenge a fourteen-year old but I half regretted that we had agreed to come.

February 15th

We had a really good evening and Chris was happy to be left with the dog and a stack of videos. When we got back after midnight he was still awake and starving! We were all up early the next day because Dougal, and Katie's Father, had to be in school for classes by 8.45. Chris joined us for breakfast. He had been unable to sleep at all and had been awake the whole night. What is happening to him?

February 22nd

Although there seem to be treatments that people have found useful for ME I feel incapable of following up any of the suggestions since no treatments have been proven and I am scared of making Chris worse. At the Cross-Party meeting Dr Mason Brown gave a presentation showing how the blood perfusion of the brain is adversely affected in ME. He treats it by using a drug called nimodipine so as to improve the circulation, but this has not yet had official sanction for use in ME.

How does the Doctor know that you have ME or CFS?

CFS is an illness characterised by unexplained fatigue lasting six months or more. The condition is not alleviated with rest and is accompanied by at least eight case-defining symptoms including sore throat, tender lymph nodes, impaired memory and concentration, myalgia or muscle pains, arthralgia or joint pains, unrefreshing sleep, post-exertional malaise (feeling ill), and headaches. Diagnosis is through the exclusion other conditions that present with similar symptoms.

The study and clinical management of CFS is complicated by the lack of biomarkers and pathogenomic signs or recognised tests for the illness. All routine tests prove to be clear.

CFS is characterised by the involvement of the endocrine (or hormone) and neuroendocrine systems, psycho-social and immune factors. A large body of research supports the link between the immune dysregulation and CFS.

February 26th

We were invited to Sunday lunch by a couple who had done voluntary work in Bosnia. I really wanted to go, especially as we had been involved in some fund-raising during the conflict; Alex had even thought of joining one of their organisation's convoys of food lorries. Chris was ensconced in front of the television. When Alex and I passed through the room to go and change, Chris called me back. "Mum," he said, "do you have to go?" He told me that, once again, he had had great difficulty in falling asleep; having gone to sleep at around three he had then only slept for five hours. He had never asked this before. If a fourteen-year old asks you to stay with them how ill must they be feeling? Alex drove away while I rang to make my apologies. I was expecting some incomprehension or at least a touch of sarcasm. I would have been incredulous myself if someone said that they were unable to leave a teenager, but she accepted it as if it were an everyday occurrence, and left me relieved and grateful.

It is beginning to dawn on me that, while it lasts, this illness is going to affect our lives. No longer will Chris be able to come home to Galloway each weekend as we used to when he was at school. The journey from Edinburgh with its two hours of twisting road is too exhausting for him. It will only be worth the effort if he comes down for more than a week.

I am looking for someone to come and be with him while I am at work, as I can not always rely on friends. I can not ask people to cover just because I want a social life. To be honest I am not too bothered about a social life while Chris is so ill.

February 27th

My sister-in-law Henny has sent me an article about a woman called Joan Copley who is forty-three years old and who was wheelchair bound with ME for five years. She had been taken to hospital with a high temperature and abdominal pains. She was then prescribed Doxycycline and felt better within 72 hours. Six weeks later she was having physiotherapy before returning to work. Doxycycline is used for acne, chest infections, and pelvic inflammatory disease. Tempting as it is to look for a cure, I feel that if this was the magic potion every patient needed, it would be prescribed. Chris has been prescribed a lot of anti-biotics and they never helped. In fact some of the literature says that they may increase a person's susceptibility to develop ME.

February 28th

I feel certain from all that I have now read that Chris has ME. I have recently been thinking about the first time Chris was ill with similar symptoms. When he was four years old there was an occasion when he had woken me every half an hour throughout the night by screaming. He was not suffering from nightmares but from a high temperature. (It is possible that the coverings of his brain were inflamed which is one explanation given for this sort of crying.) For approximately eight or nine weeks afterwards he had been lethargic and pale with a loss of appetite. During this time he had an x-ray and blood tests but they had all proved negative. I remember this curious childhood illness in particular because of a conversation in the local shop which was run by a friend.

"What on earth are you doing bringing Chris in the pushchair?" she asked me. Her shop was only half a mile from our house and we regularly walked the distance.

I had answered, "Chris simply can't walk this far."

Eventually, because Chris was eating nothing except the occasional boiled sweet, the doctor ordered special supplement drinks. Suddenly, just before we had to try them, he was better.

> Is the brain involved in ME?
>
> Cognitive problems, or the mental processes of the brain, are commonly reported in persons with CFS and are one of the most frequent and disabling symptoms associated with this disorder.
>
> In a study of fifty papers between 1988 and 2008 Cockshell reported that the main areas found to have cognitive defects were in the domains of attention, memory and reaction time. Deficits were not apparent on tests of fine motor speed, vocabulary, reasoning and global functioning (how well a person is meeting various problems in daily living).
>
> CFS patients showed moderate to large impairments in simple and complex information processing speed in tasks requiring working memory over a sustained period of time.
>
> A small but significant group were affected in a test of memory for figures.

March 1st

We are waiting for an appointment to see Dr Speight, the consultant paediatrician at Durham Hospital. Our GP has had this appointment authorised by our Health Board because there is no-one in this area who is particularly conversant with ME.

March 2nd

Last year a group of four of Chris' school friends used to come back to the flat with him on Thursdays. School finishes a little earlier that day. They have time to kill before their regular buses or trains, and I was at work. They have continued to do so. Today I was at home and had to tell them that he was unable to see anyone as he was not well enough. I had a chance to thank them for calling in and to tell them how important their visits were. I asked them call again next week. A great crowd of them had called in last Saturday but it had been too much for him and he was left bewildered and drained afterwards. Danny, Chris' particular friend, tends to come in on his own and more regularly. This week he brought some schoolwork for Chris.

March 5th

Chris still has not attempted any school work. One teacher arranged for his German class to send a card. It is the only card he has received. People do not send cards for chronic conditions. It seems that they are only for broken bones and operations and illnesses from which you will probably get well anyway. I feel very sad for him.

March 6th

Our appointment with Dr Speight in Durham is tomorrow. Chris is really bad, sweating so much that he is changing his clothes four times in a day. He is not wanting to eat and is listless and finding any occupation an effort.

March 7th

All night I kept waking up worrying. If we take Chris to Durham he will get worse. If we don't go to Durham how will we get a diagnosis? When Alex woke I told him that we could not take Chris with us, the risk was too great.

"How can we go to Dr Speight and not take Chris? We would lose the support of the entire medical profession if we don't keep this appointment." I knew Alex was right, but I also dreaded that the seven hours in the car, added to the time spent in the hospital, would make Chris even more ill. It was this hideous thought that had kept me awake. It is a bizarre concept, to see a doctor, especially a consultant who has agreed to see a patient from outside his area, and not take the patient.

"If Dr Speight really does understand ME, he will understand why we can't bring Chris." I threw out a challenge as I felt so sure that I was right.

"All right, I'll ring. And if he does agree, who is going to look after Chris?" Everything was becoming rather tense. "I'll ask Gran." I said. His Gran said that of course she would come at once. She is eighty-odd but she was prepared to jump into her car and come all the way from Ayrshire without a qualm. Then Alex rang the hospital. Dr Speight himself answered the phone and agreed to see us without Chris. So we set off, before Gran arrived, in order to be there for our one o' clock appointment.

"You seem to have made your own diagnosis," Dr Speight remarked after Alex had spoken for about ten minutes giving an outline of Chris' history. "Once the tests have been done and come back clear, which is always the case, the diagnosis is done on the history. You do not necessarily need to see the patient," he explained. I had my synopsis with me and after listening for a short while he summarised with a graph. "Is it like this?" he asked. He drew a series of tall rectangles indicating remissions and relapses, the times that Chris was well and the times that he was ill. He then followed these by drawing a series with shorter intervals and with the height slowly lowering from the norm each time. "So, he never recovered to his previous level of energy?" It was a pattern he knew. I explained that even from the age of eleven he seemed to have less energy than his friends. Dr Speight summed up by concluding that Chris' illness, the prodrome, had indeed been that episode when he was four years old and I had had to put him back in his pushchair. He thought, however, that the trigger or stressor had been the burglary.

"When Chris returns to school he must not do sport for at least six months." He then told us about one child who was sporty, like many of them are, and who had recovered enough to return to school. Unfortunately a well intentioned and enthusiastic P.E. teacher had said to him, 'Why don't you try just one session?' The boy relapsed for six months. In another case a girl was doing well at University when she decided to travel across America in her summer holiday. She never got back to University.

He gave us a small handout. "I'm a therapeutic nihilist when it comes to ME" he said.

"Plenty of Tender Loving Care, but I have no remedy. I use melatonin to try and help the sleep. I find that once the sleep pattern returns you tend to begin to see some recovery. It is important that everyone around him understands." He explained his belief that there were no interventions, but that care, time and just allowing the child to get better was the best healing recipe.

He went on to tell us about a girl who had been sent from doctor to doctor trying to diagnose her illness. Finally the considered opinion was that she had phobias that she was failing to address. Her Mother took her to a lecture by Dr Speight. At the end of the lecture, sitting at the back in her wheelchair, he discovered that the girl was crying. "Is it something I've said?" he asked. "No", answered her Mother, "it's just that finally she knows what's the matter with her."

Dr Speight then spoke mainly to Alex, explaining that there was a report to be published soon by the Chief Medical Officer in England. It was to decide under which category ME (which is also called Chronic Fatigue Syndrome), would fall. It seems that there is a strong lobby to re-categorise ME under Mental Health. Dr Speight's own career and credibility is at stake if this is the outcome. He has diagnosed around 200 children and is unsure what his position would be if ME was defined as a mental condition. The review is to be published in January 2002. Alex seemed to understand the implications. We arrived home at around 7 pm.

What is the CMO report?

In 1998 the Chief Medical Officer commissioned a report on the situation in the UK of CFS/ME. It was published in 2002.

In his introduction he says that CFS/ME is a genuine illness 'which imposes a considerable burden on the health of the UK population. The disbelief and controversy over CFS/ME that exists within the profession has done nothing to dispel public disbelief.' The report was limited by the lack of good quality research.

March 8th

I rang the school absence line again. You are meant to ring in every day, but I left a message to say that I would let them know what was happening each week. It's a good thing that we have a diagnosis or I'm sure someone would be querying why Chris is not yet back at school. Some of Dr Speight's case histories are alarming. If a school is unsympathetic they start investigating non-attendance thinking that the child could be school-phobic. Some children have even been removed from their parents, the perception being that the parents' influence is prolonging the illness. It is a rare psychiatric condition that involves the exaggeration or fabrication of illnesses or symptoms in a child by a primary carer. Typically the perpetrator feels satisfied by gaining the attention and sympathy of doctors and nurses. Diagnosis is difficult but the first suggested sign to look for is multiple medically unexplained symptoms. It is easy to see why ME might fall under this category should a doctor be both suspicious and mystified.

Dr Speight has had to go to court on behalf of these families because removal of the child from the parent is the only way of proving this diagnosis. Fortunately he has managed to prevent court orders in most cases where he has been convinced that the child is suffering from ME. He himself has heard someone comment 'Mothers even give up their work to look after their children.' It is hard to see how any Mother can get the balance right since they can equally easily be criticized for returning to work.

March 13th
I have sent the tape about ME made by Dr Mason Brown to my Mother.

"Have you listened to it?" she asked me on the phone last night. I told her that I hadn't. "It's rather depressing," she commented.

So I don't think I'll listen to it at the moment.

March 22nd
Chris thinks that he'll feel better in Galloway and I have managed to take some days off so that we can spend a month at home. I will go up to Edinburgh on the days that I need to and ask his Gran or someone to come and be with him. On the whole Alex is just too busy. Alex and I bought Chris his own television with a video player a few weeks ago. It was done reluctantly because it underlines the fact that we are resigned to a long haul. To transport him from Edinburgh or back again, with his television, his pillows, duvet, Play Station, games and box of videos, all of which he needs to survive, is a major upheaval.

The journey was really hard on Chris. For the first half-an-hour he was really excited and alert, after all he's not been out of the flat, and barely out of his room for nearly six weeks. After a while he went quiet and held his head in his hands. I only appreciated on the journey how much muscle work is required to negotiate all those bends and how the sunlight upsets his eyes..

April 1st
I have made a decision only to contact people whose children have had ME and have recovered. The mother of Emma (the girl that I had heard about on the station platform three years before) wrote to me in answer to my letter asking for advice. She says that it takes months to get better.

She wrote that they had to make Emma walk every day. So each day she walked to the paddock to see her horse. This was under instruction from their doctor, as psychiatrists believe that graded exercise (GET) and cognitive behavioural therapy (CBT) is the best treatment. This treatment regime means that the patient gradually increases their exercise regardless of how they feel. It also includes therapy for changing the way a person thinks which can help them feel better. Emma is now at University. I know Chris thinks he'll be back to school after the summer and is prepared to be patient. However at the rate Chris is going it could take two years!

I can't really see the point of forced exercise. When a child is moderately ill and exercise makes them worse, surely any exercise when they are this sick is not going to make them better. I can't believe that staying in bed, even for weeks, is going to mean that Chris will never be able to take exercise again. There are many examples of people, for a variety of reasons such as glandular fever, having months in bed, and they recover. Not walking is not going to perpetuate the condition and might well shorten it. Besides, we tried the 'fresh air and exercise' approach for years and it made no difference.

April 3rd

Chris is still awake most of the night and falls asleep in the early hours, or even during the day. He can never sleep for more than five hours, and he seems to be on a twenty-five hour clock. It is called 'sleep reversal' and is a recognised symptom of ME. Apparently sleep upset is the rule in ME. The sleep reversal is a disruption of the usual rhythm which regulates normal sleeping and waking patterns. Chris hates it when his sleep pattern shifts so that he is asleep from 5pm to 10pm, because he then misses out on seeing his Dad or anyone else and has no company when he is awake. He watches "Friends" endlessly. The two minute scenes are not only easy on his brain but the programme is a particularly effective antidote to loneliness. I also hate his twilight sleeping because he needs a meal just as I am going to bed and another around 3 am. Alex has bought me a microwave to help with this.

April 5th

Chris is still sweating and changing his socks several times a day. I have read that ME patients have spells of fidgety leg and arm movements while they are asleep, sometimes they are almost paralysed from a few seconds to even two minutes when they wake, and they can have waking dreams. Their insomnia is due to disturbances of the brain, as is their weird temperature control. Sweating and slowing of the heart rate is also common. Sometimes they feel so ill that they think that this is how you feel before you die. Chris can only manage a bath every three or four days. He came down to-day having cut his hair himself with scissors. There were tufts of hair and bald patches all over his scalp. When his Gran arrived she looked shocked. Chris is past caring.

April 6th
Helen has come to stay for two nights. She is nearly a year older than Chris and is an outgoing teenager with a sense of fun and she makes us laugh.

"Are you going to leave me with that?" she asked, indicating Chris, who looks as if he has come out of Bedlam. She was unperturbed and Chris enjoys her company. I hardly had to explain ME to her since her brother has a friend with it.

"It's to do with the immune system, isn't it?' Helen commented. 'It's a good thing I have got rid of my cold." Helen is a diabetic and is more than usually aware what infections can do to her own, as well as to others' bodies. I am impressed by her understanding and find her ability to take his illness at face value strangely relaxing. As far as she is concerned Chris is ill and I do not need to elaborate.

April 22nd
It is Chris' 15th birthday to-day. Iain and Dougal have given him a mobile phone so that he can keep in touch with his friends. He has asked me to buy him a mini-discman from a shop in Chambers Street with his birthday money when we return to Edinburgh.

April 23rd
I have decided to follow the school term and, in order to keep some structure to this life that has none, we have come back to Edinburgh. Chris is aware that his friends are unlikely to call in during the holidays even if he were in Edinburgh, and if we come to Galloway it stops him from feeling so lonely.

April 27th
Chris' Housemaster called in this evening to see if Chris would be able to go to Carbisdale Activity Centre with his year after the exams. He told me that they find that the week of outward bound activities forms a significant part of the boys' educational development, and was

very anxious for Chris to join them. I cannot give him an answer. It seems unlikely that Chris will be well enough, but we still hope for a miracle. Although I know that in the light of Dr Speight's advice a week of physical exercise is totally out of the question so soon after being ill. I still cannot bring myself to dampen Chris' hopes by an outright 'No'. I am finding the prospect of a prolonged illness sadly daunting as well. I fear that if I said 'no' now it might tempt fate and it might become a self-fulfilling prediction.

May 5th

Last night I spent two hours with Chris before finally going to bed after midnight. When he hasn't had much sleep (he woke at 10.30 am having only got to sleep at 6.30 am) he is so tired that anything is too much effort. He has been changing his clothes two or three times a day for the past two days because he has been sweating so much. It's a strange sticky sweat.

May 7th

I asked Chris to let me treat his head. I was hoping that perhaps it might help with his sleep, and since I have practised my physiotherapy mobilisations on his skull before he was ill, he submitted with only a little reluctance. I may be reading things into my palpation but his skull felt small, and tight. It is so frustrating to be able to help so many other people and be unable to do anything to help your own son.

May 8th

I have been buying Lego for Chris to do and to begin with he enjoyed it, and it certainly helped him to pass the time. Recently however I have found him agitated, and pouring with sweat, and then telling me that a piece was missing or that the instructions didn't make sense. He is now playing a game of flicking cards into a pot. This is a game that he learnt from watching "Friends". I just do not know how we would have survived the last months without "Friends"; when everyone is asleep, at least they are there. The other way of passing the time at the moment seems to be these tedious Play Station games. To me they are quite mindless, but they do not tax his brain too much and that is probably why they suit him. Possibly they allow him to relax. I haven't delved into any reasons for his symptoms, since at present we are clinging on by our finger tips. It is, none the less, a terrible waste of time. Time that we could both be spending differently. Our time is just spent waiting for Chris to get better.

How does a doctor know if you have ME?
Why a specific name is needed for this disorder

Dr E.D. Acheson was the Chief Medical Officer from 1984-1991. He was also an early researcher into ME. In 1959 he studied fourteen epidemics that had broken out worldwide.

He wrote that ME needed a specific name because it had a specific identity. Recognition of an illness depends on its clinical pattern and be sufficiently characteristic to separate this disorder from other conditions. Dr Acheson felt that ME fulfilled this criteria.

The importance of a clinical entity, or the ability to recognise Benign Myalgic Encephalomyelitis, Icelandic Disease, or Epidemic Neuromyasthenia as different from any similar disease that is already recognised, is that otherwise 'the syndrome will become a dumping ground for non-specific illnesses characterised by fluctuating aches and pains, fatigue and depression', especially in sporadic cases where the physician may not be familiar with the disease now known as CFS.

Characteristics:-

The incubation period appeared to be between four days and six weeks.

The prodrome, or initial illness, was usually abrupt with headache and muscle pain, fever rarely more than 100F with nausea, back and neck stiffness and sensory disturbances were the most common symptoms. These complaints and the malaise that accompanied them were out of proportion to the fever which sometimes was absent.

The mental symptoms which are a constant feature of all outbreaks are not typical of hysteria. Shallowness and belle indifference were not seen. Depression and undue emotional lability were the rule in the acute stage and during convalescence, along with impairment of memory,and difficulty in concentration. These symptoms are more consistent with brain damage than with hysteria.

Relapses have been a feature of all but one of the fourteen outbreaks studied. In women the relapses tended to coincide with their menstrual periods. Physical exertion and cold weather were other contributing factors. Relapses mainly occur within three months but some have suffered a second attack up to three years later. Relapses can consist of the same or new symptoms, and can be much worse. Of those who had recovered only a small per cent were completely free of symptoms.

It was significant that Gilliam's account of the 1934 outbreak in Los Angeles was that later accounts had no knowledge of this study yet their observations were very similar. Gilliam wrote that the average period of illness until return to work was 13.5 weeks, yet half of his patients were still on the sick list. In Durban the moderate cases returned to work within 3-4 months. In the Royal Free a period of six weeks convalescence was needed for patients who had been in bed for one month and even they could only return to a four hour working day.

May 9th

Dr Speight is speaking at the Cross-Party group to-morrow. We only told Chris today that afterwards Dr Speight will be coming to the flat to see him. Dr Speight has to see him to confirm his diagnosis. Chris does not want to see him, or any doctor for that matter, even although he knows that Dr Speight believes in ME. Dougal has thoughtfully arranged for his cricketing friend, Damien, who is a 'pro' over from Australia, to come and be with Chris so that Alex and I can both go to the meeting. We hope that having Damien for company will give him something to look forward to.

May 10th

Dr Speight spent ten minutes alone with Chris, no more. He told us during a brief chat on his way out that he had impressed upon Chris the dangers of returning to sport until he was fully well.

When Damien had gone we went through to Chris' room. Damien had decided to give Chris his Tigers top as a present. Chris was wearing it over his sweatshirt. He did not look as delighted as I had hoped by Damien's visit and it was not until he and I were alone later that I discovered why. He had got up and was looking out of the window. He spoke with his back to me.

"I won't be able to play cricket for three years, will I?"

I hesitated. He turned round to face me.

"I won't, will I?" He insisted. "If I go back to school next year and then have to wait a year before playing sport? What will I *do* in the summer?"

May 12th

This is an awful week and any recovery that we had gained was lost when Chris realised that Dr Speight really was coming to see him despite his wish to the contrary. Alex eventually persuaded Chris that we were not going to change our minds about the decision. We had no choice but we hadn't reckoned on this reaction.

Even though this has been traumatic it could have been so very much worse. I hear stories of people who were hounded back to school, not believed, sent to psychiatrists, or sent from doctor to doctor. At least with the advice we were lucky enough to receive from Dr Vance Spence at that first Cross-Party meeting Chris has been spared too many consultations or conflicting opinions. Dr Speight is almost the only paediatric consultant with any expertise on the subject of ME, and we were fortunate to be in the right place at the right time, and to have a GP prepared to refer us. It is all a matter of chance.

2001 Summer

"O aching time, O moments big as years"

John Keats

Chris had been ill, seriously ill, unrelentingly and with no good spells or even good days, for five months. Apart from glandular fever I had heard of no-one who had had a child ill for so long unless they were undergoing chemotherapy. This was not how I envisaged ME. To feel ill all the time and to see no hint of improvement. If he had glandular fever I would begin to see signs of recovery by now. The days repeated themselves and in the background questions would appear and reappear. What should or should he not do? If he began to feel better should I put the reins on, or allow him to do what he wanted?

We were to learn from experience that ME does not allow the luxury of utilising a good day without extracting its revenge. How should we progress? By allowing nature to take its course and follow Dr Speight's 'therapeutic nihilism', or risk some form of treatment? Chris eventually felt so poorly that he indicated that something had to be done. The question was what should we do when there was the potential for treatments to make him worse? Finally there was the question of education. The contact with teachers could reduce his isolation. If his brain was unable to function, however, would lessons overtax him or leave him depressed at his lack of achievement? More importantly could attempting school work actually make his ME worse? Over the next six months most of these questions were tackled, and as there were no guidelines, I had to make the decisions.

May 13th
Jane, a friend and fellow physiotherapist, rang to see about the outcome of Dr Speight's visit.

"Why is Chris always worse after he has seen a doctor?" Jane observed as we talked; she remarked that the same downturn in his health had followed our visit to the previous consultant.

I told Jane that we have been trying double melatonin, on Dr Speight's advice, to try and help with Chris' sleep, but that he can't bear the smell of the tablets. He can smell them even when I am at the end of the bed. It's unbelievable! I think we will have to stop the tablets, as we can see no improvement; he becomes upset each time he has to take one. He is also taking selenium, on the advice of a well-wisher who sent a whole folder on selenium deficiency to Alex.

May 14th

This is a peculiar disease. Nothing can prepare you for it. If your child is ill you sit and do things with them. Suddenly, you are faced with the opposite problem. Now stimulation beyond his capacity makes Chris worse and his capacity is so restricted that the only course of action is inactivity. Jane asked me what we do each day. How do you pass the time doing nothing? Mostly Chris just wants me to be there. I can't read, it seems wrong somehow, and since the curtains are closed it is too dark to do so. Chris needs me there almost as if I were going through this with him. Our routine varies little from day to day, although the order varies depending on Chris' sleep time. If he falls asleep around 3.30 or 4.30 in the morning it means he doesn't need me until after 10am and I can go out to do some shopping or make some phone calls. I keep the phone on silent so that no-one can ring in, until he wakes. His sleep quality is poor and lasts only five hours so that he wakes unrefreshed and groggy and it takes some time before he emerges to go to the bathroom.

I cook him some sausages and cut them into chunks so that he can eat them with a fork while watching the T.V., and I'll take a cup of coffee and sit with him.

Chris might ask me to change a video for him and once I hear a few chuckles I take his plate, refill his glass of squash and add some sweets and biscuits to the tin of 'emergency' rations. Then I am free to go and do a few essential household chores.

If he decides to have a bath I'll run the water for him and take the chance to change his bed or hoover his room. He cannot bear the noise of the hoover, and it is a conundrum how to keep the rest of the flat clean. I give him a fresh supply of t-shirts, he wears two or three on top of each other with a sweat-shirt on top, and a clean pair of pyjama bottoms.

I'll have my lunch with him, although he rarely has his at the same time. Chris might play one of his endless Play Station games. There is one in particular which is set in Japan. It seems to consist of going from one bleak room to another. Despite never reaching the final objective, it succeeds in passing hours of his time. I might do some tapestry, (knitting is too irritating with its clicking needles), angling the lamp almost on top of my lap so as to reduce the effect of the light.

In the afternoon I might offer to find him a new magazine or go for some sweets. The Tymes' Trust (The Young ME Society) suggest that you try and provide one treat each day. Sometimes I'll make krispies, or ask what new video he would like to hire.

May 15th

I have arranged Chris' room so that it is like a bed-sit and more comfortable for his friends. I have also propped up a piece of hardboard onto an old table and attached a dart board. The landlady would throw us out if she knew. He had his first game this evening when Alex came home. It lasted about fifteen minutes. Chris sat down when it was his Dad's turn to throw. Alex had to retrieve all the darts!

> Poliomyelitis and ME
>
> In poliomyelitis the virus attacks the anterior horn cells or posterior horn cells in the spinal cord and attacks **efferent** outgoing or 'doing' nerves. In severe cases paralysis of muscles is obvious. In ME it is thought that viruses have a propensity to attack **afferent** incoming or 'feeling' nerves. The effect is more noticeable to the patient than the doctor. Mutual antagonism between poliomyelitis and other members of the group is well known. Where poliomyelitis has been raging in the population ME is also often found. Although the virus has not been identified, when samples from ME patients were injected into monkeys, minute red spots were found along the sciatic nerves. Infiltration of the nerve roots with lymphocytes and monocytes and patchy damage to myelin sheaths (coverings of the nerves) was seen, and one of the monkeys died.

May 16th

Alex and I have supper together most evenings when he is up in Edinburgh but tonight Chris' routine coincided with ours so we all ate in his room. Before I went to bed I called in to say goodnight and to have a chat and to make sure he had everything he needed for the long night. He is not falling to sleep until around 4 am and I suggested he telephoned

Iain if he wanted to. If he rings around midnight or even later, because America is five hours behind us, it breaks up the long vigil, and also relieves me from checking him until after two or three in the morning.

May 17th

I was half way through my session at work this morning when Alex rang through to the Clinic. Chris had rung him because he had the shakes and was upset and frightened. My colleagues said that they would cover for me and that I could leave at once. I ran to the taxi rank and was at the flat within twelve minutes. I think Chris was short of food because he soon recovered but he gave me, and himself, a scare. I realise that I will have to find someone to cover for my Monday sessions. I need to make sure that he is given his breakfast, whatever time he wakes.

May 20th

Today there has been a curious sequel to the drama earlier in the week. At the Clinic we had to reschedule the appointment of the teenage dancer whose session I had to leave. At the start of our session I apologised to the young dancer and her Mother and explained a little about Chris and his illness. At the end of the session the Mother asked, "Excuse me, but what did you say about his curtains being closed all the time?" I answered that I had said that it was a bit depressing as he always keeps his curtains closed because the light hurts his eyes.

An extraordinary look came over her face as if she had made a connection, or had a glimmer of understanding. "Can I ring you this evening?" she asked.

Later, she told me that her daughter had been treated for behavioural problems for the last two years. Despite having three other children who had no problems, they had been given advice on parenting. She had brought her daughter to the clinic because her feet were sore when she was dancing. Her tutors had been unsympathetic and were unaware of the effort and pain that she endured in order to continue her dancing. She had repeated fungal infections as well as pain. These and many of her other symptoms, it transpired, resembled Chris'. To find out more, and to see if this might be the case, I suggested that she contact Dr Mason Brown.

May 21st

Danny and the other Thursday friends called in after school again.

Once they had seen themselves out Chris told me that Danny had been looking on the Internet to find out about ME.

Danny told them that he had read that some people do not believe in it. "I said to myself, 'Oh no, here we go!'" Chris related. He saw my face change from interest to concern and then said with a grin. "But Danny said 'we believe in it, because we've seen it!'" This is a huge relief.

May 24th

Chris has 'burning skin'. It dawned on me that it could be a reaction to the amytriptylene. Amytriptylene is a psychoactive drug which is commonly used for major depression but small doses are given for insomnia. Chris has been taking it instead of melatonin for the past ten days. I will suggest to Chris that he stops it. There has been no change in his sleeping pattern anyway and I dislike the thought of these drugs. I am very wary of drugs, in any form, for ME.

May 25th

This week his 'year' are at the Carbisdale Activity Centre. Chris is a bit down especially as today is Thursday and his friends usually visit. It's difficult to know what to do to fill the gap. I bought him a new video to watch this afternoon. I never thought that I would use the television as a 'baby-sitter' but I feel easier if I know he is entertained especially when I am at work. Chris worries about all the magazines and videos that I have been buying him. Already, his video collection is impressive and it does seem a lot as the collection builds up. If he was ill for a week it would seem quite reasonable to buy a couple of videos and a magazine but, somehow, it doesn't when an illness goes on for months. The rationale is the same but he thinks he looks spoiled. I try to tell him that it is just a change of emphasis. It is arguably a reasonable use of our money when he has had no need of new clothes, does not wear shoes, go out or play sports.

May 28th

Dougal arrived down from Perth again this Friday. Although he works in Perthshire he plays cricket with a local club at weekends. He has offered to stay with Chris so that I can go to Galloway to do some work. I seem to be constantly asking him and his friends to help out. It is so much better for Chris to have younger people around, but on the other hand he can easily become exhausted and it is only with me that he can recover. It is a juggling act.

May 31st

I spoke to Iain today. He sounded tired, unusual for him, perhaps work and the heat are taking their toll. He also has a sort of hay fever. He asked me. "Mum, does Chris have to ring every night? Half the time I just don't know what to talk about." It had relieved my mind enormously when I went to bed to know that Chris could call Iain. I felt a bit guilty but I told Iain that he had no idea what a life-line he had been. Chris can talk to Iain about the films he's been watching and he really doesn't want to talk only to me. This disease is making demands on both Iain and Dougal as well as Alex and myself.

June 1st

Gran suggested to Chris that his feet would be warmer if he wore shoes instead of socks, but he told her they were too heavy. He uses plastic cutlery instead of that provided in the flat because it is lighter. He doesn't wear a watch and when someone sent him a wrist magnet to see if it would help that was too heavy too.

I notice that Chris is not cleaning his teeth. When I broached the subject he said he couldn't be bothered, he has to sit on the edge of the bath to do them and it is a huge effort. I'll see if an electric toothbrush will help. I notice that when Chris says he can't be bothered he means that he has not the energy.

June 3rd

Since stress of any kind makes him worse, I have adopted a policy of saying that nothing matters, and that nothing is any trouble or any effort. Today he upset lucozade over the laptop that his Aunt has lent him; that really was a problem, but we made light of it. After a while this mantra becomes true. I am not doing much except looking after him anyway and if fetching something or changing a video or finding a computer repair shop for him helps, then it is really not a problem.

June 8th

When I returned to part-time work a year after Chris was born I had asked a retired couple, Jean and Jimmy, of whom I was very fond, to look after Chris for one day a week. They remained good friends as he got older, even looking after him if he had days off school, until we left the village. They have come over for the weekend so as to be with Chris, because I have to be on hand for the dance students who are performing their end of year show. Jimmy and Chris made an airfix model. With some of his carers Chris can relax, but with others he feels he has to entertain them and I am only beginning to distinguish the two groups.

> Are there any studies on CFS in children?
>
> In Dundee two studies have been completed which focus on children. The first looked at 25 CFS children and compared their quality of life to 23 healthy children. They also compared their quality of life with children with diabetes type I and asthma. Of the 25 CFS children the illness had started with an infection in 88% and only one child was able to attend full-time schooling.
>
> All children were asked questions on their social limitations, pain, general well being and physical functions. In these categories the CFS children were worse than children from the other three groups, and rated themselves roughly half as well as their healthy controls.
>
> There were no differences, however, between children with CFS and healthy children in how well the family got along, or in the children's perception of their own behaviour.
>
> When looking at abnormalities in their blood and in their blood pressure and the elasticity of their arteries they found the following:-
>
> High levels of oxidative stress (shown as raised levels of isoprostanes)
>
> Reduced levels of vitamin C and E
>
> A greater percentage of white blood cells undergoing apoptosis (programmed cell death)
>
> A trend towards artery wall stiffness.
>
> Dr Kennedy who conducted the study thinks that the white blood cells are releasing an excessive amount of highly reactive free radicals possibly from exercising muscles. Increased apoptosis may be caused by a number of factors including a persistent viral infection or an abnormal immune response. 'The link between infection and apoptosis has not been proved but the finding is tantalising.'

June 16th

Curtains are drawn all the time. We are trying more salads and not having chocolate because his stomach cramps are quite sore at times. Chris also suffers from restless legs which can last for up to two hours and are often the reason he cannot fall asleep. He has tried raising them onto three pillows and that must help a little because this is how I often find him lying.

June 20th

Chris had fallen asleep at 8am, and when he woke up in the early afternoon he came through to my bedroom where I was reading. He sat down on the bed opposite and looking dazed.

"I've had such an awful dream," he said, "I dreamt that I had cancer."

I expected that my reaction would be one of alarm yet I felt very calm. It was almost is if I had been waiting for him to say this, or something similar, for some time. I had been warned by Emma's mother in her letter, that 'they feel so ill that they think they are dying and no-one is telling them'.

I told him, "I know this can happen and that is why the doctors do so many tests. Although they can not tell you what is the matter with you, they can tell you that you are not dying."

What is the Ability Scale?

The Ability Scale was devised to ascertain the degree of restriction ME was imposing on a child's life. Each level of the scale describes what percentage of a normal life can be achieved.

100% is fully active in sport, a social life and in education. 95% is no symptoms at rest but the child tires easily with physical or mental effort recovering by the next day.

At 90% the child is considered to be mildly affected. In the case of a teenager they would be described as tiring easily following games or lessons. They would find a full timetable difficult and if they were to go out socialising they would need two or three days to recover. It would only just be possible for a child with 90% on the Ability Scale to take their GCSEs or Standard Grades. 80% on the Ability scale describes a child who has mild symptoms at rest which are worsened with moderate physical or mental activity; they can manage home tuition or part-time study without difficulty. By 30% the child is severely affected. Even resting they experience moderate to severe symptoms which are exacerbated following any mild physical or mental activity. By 20% they also develop weakness in arms, hands or legs. They rarely leave the house, are able to sit for short periods only and might be able to read for 10 minutes. At 0% they are being fed, sometimes by tube, washed, and are sensitive to almost everything.

June 25th

Chris is having a better spell. The graph is marked 30% to 37%. This means that he has, to quote the Ability Scale, at 40% 'moderate to severe symptoms after any activity. Spends most of the day resting. Can manage one thing a day like a friend dropping in.' He has been sleeping for eight hours and has read two short film scripts. He can't write. He tried to jot down some ideas for a film but his handwriting deteriorated after the third line and he gave up after the fifth.

Katie is coming to stay with Chris for three days so that I can go south to see my Mother. Chris is very happy. I am more than impressed that Katie has taken on this task. It is in one sense incredibly boring because you can do so little. Katie says that she does not mind because she has a lot of work to do. On the other hand you are almost a prisoner because even if you were to go out you are always clock-watching. It is lonely too. Katie cannot invite friends to the flat because it would be too much for Chris. There are not many people who could do this, nor are there many people that I would trust Chris with.

June 28th

To Galloway for the summer. I packed all Chris' stuff; he then travelled with Alex because his car has a smoother ride. The long summer ahead looks bleak. I have approached someone locally to be with Chris twice a week when I go to work, mainly to make meals for him and just to be around. I don't really mind if she just reads the papers. I have nicknamed her Cinderella because, however I look at our problems, she has had a much rougher time. He is not very pleased but his Gran cannot come over all the time and Imogen and Kate, who came and helped at Easter, now have jobs.

June 29th

It is strange that Chris has not once asked about the flight to U.S.A. He was booked on July 6th for a three week stay with Iain who had said that he could help him coach tennis to the children at the club. A few weeks ago, when I realised that he would not be well enough to travel, I decided that I had to cancel. Perhaps the thought of what might have been, of three weeks working with Iain and the fun he would have had with him and Becca, is too hard to mention. It is ironic that just when I anticipated that I would have more freedom than I have had for over twenty-five years I am now experiencing the most restrictions.

June 30th

It is extraordinary how bizarre the temperature control is in ME. It is really warm yet Chris is always cold, wearing gloves and is under a duvet. It is thought to be due to the involvement of the hypothalamus. He is not sweating so much. He says that his head is 'hot inside' and that is why he can't sleep. The 'brain fog' seems to be like small explosions in his brain and he has to catch the threads to try and keep his concentration.

July 1st

As if to reinforce the vigilance that I keep over Chris, my every waking hour has as its background hum the thought that if I can remove all stress and effort from him, I can help his recovery. There is a heartbreaking story in the paper this week. A mother and her thirteen year old son committed suicide together because she had ME and he had been sent away to boarding school despite his distress at her fatigue and helplessness. Her husband is a hospital consultant in pharmacy and his wife had been severely ill for four years.

What about Education?

It is assumed, because the ME child is lying in bed, that they can do school work even if they can not walk. Unfortunately it is the disturbances in the brain, and the brain fog or brain fatigue, that is the ME child's most disabling and distressing symptom. Often they return to school work only in the last stages of their recovery, Some school subjects are known to be more affected than others. Maths is one of the most affected by ME. Spatial awareness is also badly affected making the judging of distances difficult. (This affects sports and driving). The TYMES Trust have pioneered a home programme to enable pupils to study and take exams as and when they are able.

July 7th

Alex and I had an interview with Chris' Headmaster this afternoon. He was very understanding but somewhat pessimistic. At his previous school there had been a boy with ME who never did recover sufficiently to go back. The Headmaster said that if he is well enough to return he can rejoin at once. However, we would have to pay full fees even if he only attended part-time. The headmaster added that he would waive the term's notice either way. Regarding home tuition he intimated that it was unfair to ask any of the current teachers since their schedules were already very full. He felt sure that via the staff room some retired teachers could be contacted. We came away rather drained. The stark facts are that Chris may not be returning in the foreseeable future.

July 10th

Iain made an interesting observation about people raising awareness about ME. "Why do people always run marathons or climb mountains?" He asked. "It gives totally the wrong message. It isn't that ME people don't want to do these things." ME people are usually very highly motivated, and it is probably because of their drive that they push themselves over the limit. Iain suggested it would be more appropriate if people did nothing so as to reflect the inactivity and privation of pleasure that ME patients are suffering. Envisage a vigil with each person provided with a mat and a six-inch standard candle. Restricted to the confines of the mat, the person would have to remain there until their lit candle burnt down and was extinguished. Some, more determined, might bring a night light, others large ornamental candles, or even church candles of three inches in diameter and twelve inches tall. They would stay until the flame spluttered and died.

July 16th

Chris is walking about the house a bit. He must be at around 40% on the Ability scale. He says that he can concentrate for fifteen minutes and is reading film scripts because they are easier. His school friend Henry has just been to stay for two nights but this was not such a relaxed visit. Their friendship was based on rugby and outdoor activities and here they can only watch television together.

July 19th

Today I gave a talk on ME with the doctor at work. I tried to explain to them that ME is not depression and that exercise, which is usually given to ME patients by physiotherapists, is far from helpful, if not downright dangerous. I never felt that I was communicating the message very well.

July 22nd

The weather is gorgeous and Chris asked if he could chip golf balls around the garden. I limited him to nine balls which I collected and then would insist that he rest for an hour. Unfortunately when I was at work and his Gran was looking after him she let him play whenever he wanted. She thought that it would not hurt and that the fresh air and exercise would be good for him. It is not an unreasonable assumption and she, like the rest of us, is so desperate for him to recover. She will also remember that, before this long spell of illness, its pattern was such that he could become better almost overnight.

July 23rd

I have taken down from the wall in the kitchen the Ability scale printed by the Tymes Trust. I thought that it would encourage Chris if he could see himself getting better, he was around 10% or 15% at the beginning but is now around 40%. The trouble is that he thinks that if he does the next stage's activities he will automatically move up the scale. This is logical thinking for ordinary health problems like recovering from an operation or a broken leg, but it is an anathema in this illness where conventional rules are turned on their head.

2001 Autumn

"No sun, no moon, no dawn, no dusk,
No proper time of day."

Thomas Hood

The crux of the debate on how to manage ME centres around whether to make the child exercise, or to allow them to pace themselves and live within their own envelope of energy, or encourage them to rest. The psychiatric approach is that managing the illness by slowly introducing increased activity will ultimately see the person recover. ME sufferers themselves are wary of this because if tried too early they tend to relapse. Sometimes they relapse so severely that they never regain their former energy levels.

The ability to exercise after an illness is the result of a healing process. Thus exercise in the recovery stage of most medical conditions is beneficial. In a recent survey of exercise as a treatment for ME a few said that it was helpful, but 50% said that it makes them worse.

Exercise, when a person is fighting an infection, makes their condition worse. Research has shown that excessive exercise causes muscles to react as if they were inflamed. This would activate the immune system. In the polio epidemic in the early 1950s those who were the most severely affected, those for example who ended up in the 'iron lung', were those who during the incubation stage of the polio virus were the most active. If ME proves to be a non-resolving infection then exercise is likely to make their condition deteriorate. Doctors who accept that ME has a physical basis have issued warnings about the risk to the health of ME patients by undergoing exercise regimes. For some ME patients very little activity could be considered over exercise. It is not yet possible to state categorically when a ME patient is in a recovery stage and therefore to advise when it is safe to start exercising. Since Chris' onset of ME had been gradual and during that time trying to return to exercise had not helped him recover, I was happy to follow Dr Speight's advice that he had to rest and carefully increase his levels of activity.

August 3rd

At last I am allowed to go outside the garden for a walk. The fields below the house have been out of bounds owing to the foot-and-mouth epidemic which started before lambing time. It is bad enough being imprisoned, so to speak, in the house but not being able to go for a walk except along the main road has emphasised our isolation. Today I just went around the perimeter of the field down by the river. I picked one of every flower and grass that I came across and counted thirty-three varieties. I showed them to Chris but I don't think that he was very impressed. The foot-and-mouth crisis has caused Alex to be so busy that I don't think he really minds the amount of time that I have to spend looking after Chris.

August 5th

This is not a good spell. Chris is sitting with his feet up all the time again and his sleep is haywire. He did manage to join us for a short while for a meal when his cousins were here, but that is all. It is awkward trying to pretend that life is unchanged when friends come and stay, even if, as one relative said they "just treat him as normal." Our life is so obviously abnormal it is hardly a wonder that very few people come to see us. He has slipped down to 30% on the Ability scale.

August 8th

Neal has been to stay for two days. He and Chris just watched films but it was great to see Chris enjoying some company. Neal is a particularly 'laid back' lad with an easy charm so I enjoy having him around as much as Chris does. Because his friends never question why Chris is as he is, I am much happier when the young are around. It probably isn't true that most people are on the whole sceptical of Chris' illness, but I can't help but feel that he and I are under scrutiny.

August 12th

Jane is here to keep me company. Chris complains that she speaks so loudly but we both value her ebullient nature and constant searches for remedies or cranky presents. I told Jane that I had had another ME case at work.

"Another case of ME at work? Do you have ME written across your forehead? What happened?" she said incredulously.

I had been treating a forty year old man for a knee problem when he suddenly looked up and asked, "Do you know anything about ME?"

I was so surprised that I stopped whatever work I was doing and answered, "Yes, my son has ME!"

He went on to say "My daughter, who is sixteen, has it. What do you think about exercise. Will it help?"

I told him that I understood that it made sufferers worse and that we had been advised to delay any exercise until they had been back to school for at least six months.

"Oh," replied the father, and he looked crestfallen, "two years ago my daughter was recovering well - she had then been ill for two years. But she was sent for graded exercise and now she is worse than she had been the first time that she was ill."

What is Deconditioning? Is fatigue in ME due to deconditioning?

Deconditioning is the word used to describe the condition of a person who has been inactive for a considerable length of time. Muscles weaken due to prolonged or enforced rest and as a result they tire easily and the person feels fatigued.

Studies as early as 1991 have shown that patients with ME have malfunctions in their muscles of a unique nature. Even relatively well ME patients, those who can take some form of exercise, suffer from muscle fatigue which has a delayed onset of up to three days later. Patients with the severer forms of ME will have a level of deconditioning, but the supposition that fatigue in ME is due to deconditioning is the reasoning behind the programme of Graded Exercise Therapy.

August 17th

The mother of the seventeen-year-old dancer made an appointment with Dr Mason Brown. She telephoned me to say that her daughter has ME. He said that she is only functioning at 60% on the Ability scale.

August 26th

The holidays seem endless and at the moment particularly joyless. I think Chris finds it easier to cope when he knows that everyone is at school. It is true there is more chance of seeing his friends in term time but also the contrast between their lives and his is not so great. I have been trying to think of a way to cheer Chris up during the next October break. I have rung Iain and he has agreed to come over for a week.

August 28th

When I told Chris about our plan he was, curiously, upset and really low for two days.

I never did discuss why and can only conjecture the cause. All our family associate Iain with activity and fun. He is a fund of ideas, many of them zany, and Chris must be aware how different everything will be when they meet this time.

September 2nd

Return to Edinburgh. Chris is looking forward to seeing his school friends again, even if it is just the half hour on Thursdays. He is sleeping longer at the moment sometimes from 4 am to 2 pm. He is eating mainly salads and cheese and chicken. His weight has stayed steady for the last two months. To begin with, when he was ten or eleven, he became quite plump, but early this year he became skinny and I asked him to tell me if he gets below 9 stone. He can't manage to read at the moment but has attempted a bit of maths.

September 4th

Chris' friends have called in two days running for half-an-hour each time and he has coped quite well.

Tonight I am meeting two teachers, arranged by his housemaster, who might be able to tutor. He has invited us to his flat and there really is no obligation for him to do anything.

September 5th

One of Chris' friends rang him on his mobile, asking for our home phone number. Each year the school sends a list of everyone's contact details, if they so wish. The school had not put his number on the list. This is the first time that I have seen Chris look betrayed, he seemed to sink in the middle of his body. He turned to me and said. "I'm not on the school list!" He must feel invisible, if you are not on the school list people will forget about you, and he must feel that the school has abandoned him.

Danny is coming to stay on Friday night. He is a faithful friend!

September 7th

Now we are trying Jane's new wonder potion. It is pretty disgusting, a sort of grass, I gather.

Chris' tutor came for their first geography lesson today. I had suggested at our meeting with his housemaster that we start with one subject. She and Chris sat at the table in the sitting room, and the session lasted about half an hour. Chris was non-committal, but he seemed to like her.

September 11th
American 'Twin towers' attack.

September 22nd
After the American disaster Chris had quite a reaction, being subdued and poorly for several days.

I have read that this has not been an uncommon response in ill people.

Five minutes homework today but I seemed to do most of it, and it was just a simple graph. It must be galling to sit and stare at a piece of work that you are sure that you used to find easy and to be completely stuck. Days and days go by with no alteration to our routine except perhaps a few minutes attempt at homework on one day, a visit from a friend on another day or the weekly lesson.

September 30th
Alex and I have just had a week in Corsica with family and friends. Once again, not unlike that which I experienced on my visit to London earlier in the year, I felt dislocated from real life. Several times I knew that I was somehow out of tune with the others, either trying too hard to join in or knowing that I had somehow misjudged the general mood of the group. Meanwhile Gran and Henny stayed with Chris and played a lot of scrabble, and discovered microwave pizzas.

October 2nd
Poor sleep. I had to cancel his lesson. When Chris has a bad day his habitually waxy yellow-white face looks even more bloodless and his eyes are even more puffy and heavy-lidded. Every movement is an effort. He does not raise his head as I enter the room, and any request is limited to the minimum of words. The title of a video is enough for me to know that he wants me to set it up. Changing channels with the remote control is a lethargic movement, and eating becomes an almost impossible challenge. He sits half upright supported by cushions so that he does not have to move to drink or eat and almost anything that I have to do in the room seems to upset the intense stillness that he requires.

Fortunately these really bad spells let up for short periods, enabling Chris to go to the bathroom or to rearrange his pillows. What he is never granted is the blessed relief of sleep. When he does sleep it takes an hour or two for him to drop off. He has all sorts of strategies like keeping a video running on low volume, or having music on, and hoping that the click as the tape finishes does not wake him. He is restless even as he sleeps, and if the telephone or any other disturbance wakes him, then he is unable to return to sleep and has to be resigned to another eighteen hours of wakefulness.

Why a diet? Which diet?

If a person's immune system is functioning poorly bacteria and viruses are able to increase where normally they are kept under control. One of the effects of ME seems to be that patients can have an overgrowth of candida in the gut. Candida is a bacteria and as such thrives on sugar. It has been found by nutritionalists that by depriving the candida of its nutriment it will die off. The recommended diet is one with no sugar, wheat or dairy (carbohydrates and lactose are converted into sugars by the body).

Candida is associated with leaky gut syndrome. The damaged gut walls allow toxins, microbes and particles of undigested food to pass into the blood stream to, amongst other sites, the brain. In Australia researchers have been looking at bacteria in the gut of ME patients. The latter seem to produce more lactic acid than controls, and the researchers suspect that the agent is an enterococcus or streptococcus bacteria.

October 4th
"This is the worst I've felt, ever."

Chris is monosyllabic and will barely talk to me since we came back from Corsica. He makes an effort when Alex comes in and they have their half-hour together. Is it time to do something? But what? In the summer I was given a cutting about Caroline Brownbill, an airline pilot, who cured herself of ME, 'and now wants to help others', She got steadily more ill over six months and then she lost her job. She proceeded to rest and only allowed herself to read. She read everything she could about ME. Many of the symptoms of ME are similar to candida overgrowth. Candida as a yeast transforms itself into an aggressive fungus called mycelia fungus, which develops little rootlets which attach to the stomach and intestine walls. They damage the lining of the walls and particles are allowed into the bloodstream that should not be there. The body treats these as foreign elements and they are attacked in the bloodstream. Caroline took advice on an anticandida diet combined with Mycopryl (a substance from the inside of coconuts which prevents the coconut milk from developing a fungus) and two years later she regained her health and her pilot's licence.

She called her organisation The ME Workshop, and its unique advantage over other clinics is that everything is done on the telephone. I will broach this with Chris when the time is right — in other words, when he is not feeling so furious with the world.

October 6th

Since he woke at 2 pm today and was feeling less miserable I suggested that we went to get a Play Station game. It takes half-an hour in the car. None of his friends were able to come this week because they are all now working very hard for their Highers. I felt desperate for him and I had to do something. Chris has found it so difficult to sleep, he is not eating much and his big toe is infected but at least he is back on the same footing with me again. I have even been able to discuss the ME workshop with him. Chris says he will do anything so long as I just tell him what to do.

October 9th

Yesterday Chris did a little homework with a lot of help from me. He was awake for 30 hours.

Short lesson today. Concentration poor.

October 11th

Sore tooth. Not eating much. Friends called in. Half-term starts. To Galloway.

October 13th

Chris is not eating much but he is not feeling so bad although he is getting a lot of nightmares. His tooth has cleared, thank goodness, I was dreading having to take Chris to a dentist in case the effort involved would make him worse. It's a dread that never goes away. It seems impossible to make him better but it is possible to stop him from getting worse. Or is it?

October 19th

I collected Iain from Glasgow airport at 9 am. I engineered a stop on the way back for us to have breakfast, so that I could explain what things were like now. I almost felt embarrassed as I clarified the situation and explained how gentle Iain would have to be in his interaction with his younger brother.

"You mean I can't tease him at all?" Iain was incredulous.

October 21st

Once Iain had spent time with Chris he realised how fragile he was. Fragile is the only word I can use to describe how we approach him and his condition. Sometimes he is robust enough to join in our conversations, at other times it is best to leave him quietly until he is ready. Iain and Dougal can see that doing everything for Chris is a necessity. Dougal has realised, as Iain will, how easy it is to willingly look after him. It is only because it is unnatural to look after a younger brother in this way that initially they hesitate. It is fortunate that there is such a large age gap between them. I can imaging the impact on a family where all the siblings are close in age. The healthy ones would suffer as much as the sick. Not only can they never do anything as a family, but their mother would, inevitably, be embroiled in caring for the sick child, and the others would resent it. At least Iain and Dougal being much older lead their own lives and can make allowances.

October 29th

Iain has left. I don't think it was a very exciting week for him although he had Dougal's company for a few days. I had arranged for Iain to take some wakeboard lessons to get rid of his excess energy. The loch is extremely chilly especially for someone who is spoiled by heat for most of the year. All the family acknowledge that Iain has boundless energy and he was as amused as the rest of us by Dougal's succinct summary that, of the available family energy, Iain has taken more than 50%, leaving some for him but almost none for Chris!

October 30th

Jane has sent me a cutting from the journal for GPs.

Dr Mary Church, who is also on the BMA medical ethics committee, is quoted as saying:

"Never let the patient know you think ME does not exist, never advise an ME patient to make a review appointment."

October 31st

Half-term is over.

I am tackling the instructions in ME Workshop book. It is a bit daunting because Chris has to cut out dairy products, wheat, tea, chocolate and sugar. It recommends that we make a food diary and buy ingredients such as quinoa and carob bars. However I will do what I can to begin with, depending on what Chris can bear to eat. He has stopped the haliborange because they contain sugar and instead is taking herbal Echinacea for his immune system and maximol which is a cocktail of vitamins.

The Workshop advocates relaxation and rest periods. Formal relaxation is not something that I would suggest to Chris but probably an adult would understand its efficacy. Once a person and their immediate circle of friends and family accept ME then no energy is wasted in futile efforts to 'act as normal' and this energy can then be focussed towards allowing the body to heal. The main thrust of the ME Workshop, however, is the connection between the brain and the gut. A lack of adequate nutriments being absorbed from a damaged gut means that the brain fails to receive sufficient healthy blood from which to feed its cells.

The first meal I tried was chicken Thai style with green peppers, ginger, chilli, onions and egg noodles. Everything has to be cooked in olive oil which must not be reused.

Chris said he could eat this for a year!

What is Pacing?

In a survey conducted by ME self-help groups and MEAssociation, pacing has proved the most useful method of managing ME symptoms. The nature of the illness is that patients have 'good days' and 'bad days' and the temptation is to do too much on the 'good days' resulting in unnecessarily bad 'bad days'. The pattern is called boom and bust, and it is extremely difficult for anyone to judge what is too much. Pacing is living within the person's own energy envelope and each person has to work out for themselves what is their level of activity.

Pacing is one of the management strategies researched by the confusingly named PACE trial which started in 2003.

November 2nd

"I've felt the best I've felt all week. I know by how my legs are if I'm going to be bad."

Chris has about eight pillows. He has these three very flat ones that he has under his head to sleep on or to rest his head when watching television, and five at the end of his bed to put his legs up on. Usually he sits in the bucket armchair, which must be terrible for his back, with pillows on the dressing table stool, wrapped up in a duvet. He wears pyjamas and a sweat shirt over several T-shirts, thick socks and gloves. He has taken over Alex's old farming socks and wears his black school gloves.

November 4th

I had to attend a two day course, held on the outskirts of Edinburgh, which luckily finished early each day. It is ridiculous how much I fret if I have to be away for any length of time. I just know that when I am at home Chris uses the least amount of energy; hopefully that can be used to allow his body to heal. Andy and then Julia held the fort for me.

November 8th

One of my patients, a final year medical student, asked me where I had gone on holiday this summer. I explained that it was a bit difficult at present because my son had ME. He spun round from his prone position and said, "Yes, what is ME? I don't even know what it stands for."

November 22nd

It was decided by the ME Cross-Party Group to ask Dr Allan Cumming from the Edinburgh Medical School to speak. Apparently, teaching at Medical Schools has totally changed; no longer do they learn about diseases by rote. If they show an interest in an illness or condition they are led by a tutor to explore the aetiology, pathology, treatment etc. "What if the tutor has entrenched views on the subject?" someone asked. "It could be that the tutor on ME believed that it was a somatisation disorder." In a heavy syllabus such as medical students have, is it likely that they would choose to study ME? That is assuming that they have even heard of it.

November 28th

On the whole Chris has had a poor month. He had a week of being in bed all day feeling so cold. He was been unable to see his friends and I cancelled his lessons on two occasions. He also has a sore throat. However we are persisting with the new diet. Yesterday for example he had two sausages, a rasher of bacon, and tea with sugar for breakfast.
Thai meal and chips for lunch.
Popcorn for snack and one chocolate krispie and organic fruit juice.
Burger and salad for supper.
All the meals are at weird times but we still give them the chronological names.

What about Depression and Mood changes in ME?

Twist and Maes in 2009 in Belgium have shown anomalies in ME/CFS patients in the functioning of the HPA axis (the hypothalamus area of the brain, the pituitary endocrine master gland and the adrenal gland above the kidneys loop). Studies can demonstrate a distinction between ME/CFS, burn-out and depression. The HPA axis deals with physical and emotional stress.

Reduced functioning of the HPA axis could lead to an exaggerated stress response in the areas that it regulates, namely,temperature control, digestion, immune system, mood sexuality and energy management. It is a major part of the system that controls the body's reaction to stress, trauma and injury.

Having a psychiatric disorder was not a predictor that the illness would be prolonged. Cockshell found that the majority of studies that examined the impact of self-reported depression in CFS on cognition functioning failed to find a relationship.

Those studies which categorised CFS on the basis of psychiatric diagnosis (most commonly Major Depressive Disorder and Dysthymia or Chronic Depression) found cognitive impairment was greater for people without. a co-existing psychiatric disorder than for those with a co-morbid diagnosis. Hence the cognitive problems in CFS patients are unlikely to be due to a psychiatric disorder.

November 30th

I gave Chris aspirin and stepsils for his throat.

I have read that sensitivity to drugs is virtually pathognomonic [a sign or symptom that is characteristic or unique to a particular disease] to ME and I loathe having to give him any. Luckily he missed his BCG last year because several cases of ME have been triggered by this vaccination and it could, possibly, have made him even more ill.

Chris has had a couple of better days and has invented 'football' in his bedroom. Silver paper balls on a tray. Occasionally he uses a soft ball rather like playing squash against the wall. Ever the kill joy, I beg him to limit this to a few minutes a day. Last night he slept from 11.30pm - 8am which is nice for all of us.

December 12th

Chris has relapsed again. Perhaps he is playing too much with his soft ball. He has been really low. I have decided to stop the lessons. Chris can't manage any homework. I have also stopped the Living Energy Powder which we have been trying for ten days, Chris says it makes him feel angry. His twitching legs lasted for two hours. As a distraction Alex has challenged him to stop biting his nails, with a hefty bribe.

December 13th

This evening was Helen's Christmas Carol Service and, because it took place in the church opposite the flat, I went with Jamie, her Dad. As we were leaving Jamie stopped to ask a Mother about her son who had ME. He turned to introduce me, explaining that my son had ME as well. In the brief time we had to talk she told me that they had been living in Canada and had found a diet that helped. It was similar to the ME Workshop diet. It had worked and her son was now at University. This is very encouraging considering the difficulties we are having in cutting out sugar.

December 16th

Danny, Angela and another school friend called in. They were in town because it was Saturday.

"My head rushes are happening more often, it's as if my brain stops and I have to make it work." Chris complained after they had left and then he added, "Everyone is changing. They only talk about parties."

Sleep?

Sleep disturbance is always present in ME. Various forms of sleep disturbance are experienced by ME patients. They can experience different problems at different times, or have two or three at the same time.

Some sleep excessively and have to be woken, some have insomnia, and others have sleep reversal where they sleep during the day and are awake all night. They are unable to change this voluntarily by 'sleep hygiene' or sensible regimes.

Dream disorders, leg and arm movements while asleep, and sleep paralysis can also be experienced. At night their heart rate can slow down, and their temperature control is disrupted so that they sweat profusely, both of which disrupt their sleep.

December 18th

"I dreamt they made me go out, and I took a drug that made me feel great for seven minutes, but we only went bowling."

December 20th

"I have lost eleven months. I feel as if I have woken up and it's all a dream. Mum, I can't bear it."

2002 Winter

"The night of time far surpasseth the day"

Sir Thomas Browne

ME patients believe that their illness has a physical cause, and over the last ten years research is emerging that gives credence to this view. All but a fifth of ME patients suffer from pain, and this pain is worse than that experienced by the average Multiple Sclerosis or Rheumatoid Arthritis patient. Almost all suffer from muscle cramps, twitching, acute tenderness or weakness in their extremities. In 2002 we knew of no research, and had to rely on gut instinct, and the support of a doctor if he or she could be found. Research is showing a number of abnormalities in a variety of systems in ME, in white blood cells, in muscles, in the autonomic system, in the gut and in the brain. Patients are well aware that one of the main problems in ME is cited as being that there are 'too many symptoms'. These research findings might one day explain them.

Medicine is essentially detective work; that is its fascination. It seems incomprehensible that doctors are not intrigued by ME. It is a relatively new disease, first reported in 1934, and it is an illness from which many eventually recover. It has known links with Polio (for example in Los Angeles and Iceland) and like Polio it is an endemic illness with sporadic outbreaks. Polio was conquered through an onslaught of trials by scientists.

In the meantime patients have to live from day to day and endure what the illness decides to hurl at them. This is what we experienced in 2002.

January 1st
Jane and her husband Jeremy were due to come and stay for New Year. Entertaining over Christmas, and trying to make it the same as any

other year, has proved too much. I cannot cope and am being irritable. Every night's sleep is broken. Chris is awake until 2am or 3am. I find my head feels thick and buzzes if we have company for long. Having to keep everything going, and worrying whether Chris is overexerting himself and will have a relapse, is all too much. I had to cancel. Jane was incredibly understanding.

January 2nd

This is some way to start a new year. I have spent the last two days in bed and Chris has brought up my supper!

January 12th

Cindy came to sit with Chris for the evening while we went to a charity dinner dance. Emma's mother asked me how Chris was recovering. Emma was the young equestrian who had developed ME. "There's really no change," I told her. She looked shocked. "Oh, I'm so sorry, I'm so sorry," she said. In her letter she had warned that it would take months but even she had not envisaged twelve months with no improvement. When we returned Chris and Cindy were watching the football together. They had found common ground. Cindy has been so sensitive in looking after Chris, keeping out of his way, and doing all sorts of jobs for me, aware what a teenager must feel at having to have a 'childminder'. Her patience has been rewarded.

January 17th

Everyone in the Cross-Party group is becoming anxious about the outcome of the Chief Medical Officer's report on CFS/ME. The working party has finished, but the document has not been released yet. Professor Hooper, along with two colleagues from the University of Sunderland, have published an "Information for Clinicians and Lawyers. What is ME? What is CFS?" in advance of the publication about which they have severe doubts as they fear that there will be no reference to it being an organic disease.

January 30th

The Chief Medical Officer's report has been published. It is a hugely fat document which took fifty people and three years to prepare.

There was a debate on ME in the Scottish Parliament. One journalist, who wanted a human-interest slant to the coverage, approached Alex.

Alex felt that he had to talk about Chris because this would highlight the plight of other children. They also wanted a photo of Chris. Since he has been ill Chris has not allowed us to take photos of him but Jimmy took one when they visited at Christmas, to show off his digital camera. He is able to send the photo through the Internet. As there is little likelihood of him knowing, we saw no reason to tell Chris.

January 31st

Chris' friends called in after school and brought the newspaper article in with them. They were excited to have recognised him but he was furious with us. He railed at me. "You knew I would not say yes if you had asked me, so you just did not ask," and then he refused to speak to me anymore. I had to ring Alex and ask him to come home. We could justify it, but Chris felt that we had betrayed him. We explained that there was a pressing need for people to be aware of ME because that seemed to be the only way of driving the medical profession. We argued that without a change of attitude among doctors no research or treatment would be undertaken and people would go on being ill like he was. Since Alex is convenor of the Cross-Party group, and the press had shown an interest in the first ever debate on ME in the Parliament, he had been interviewed. Naturally they needed to know why Alex had an interest in, and knowledge of, ME.

We couldn't really apologise because none of this could be undone, but, knowing that Chris would one day understand, I hoped that he would then forgive us.

February 5th

We received quite a lot of mail following the article in the newspaper. One lady wrote five pages explaining how she had weaned herself off Stematol [nausea pill], paracetomol, and prozac (for depression) by identifying what her body is allergic to by using kinesiology. She was very encouraging. Another wrote advising an aloe vera drink, another to use diet changes along with drinking copious amounts of water, yet another sent an article extolling cognitive behavioural therapy and another suggested magnets. It was overwhelming how much effort people took to try to help us and to give us heart. All of these things help different people at different times. Some people wrote to say that they had discovered that they had been suffering from something else, such as Lyme disease (usually caught from deer ticks) instead.

February 9th

The most interesting letters we have received have been from three members of a family whose daughter has now recovered from ME. The daughter wrote separately to us and to Chris. This was a particular kindness since she wanted to blank out those two years. She did not want to be remembered as 'the ME sufferer'. She said she would understand if Chris was unable to read her letter and I read it instead. When she was fourteen and unable to shower herself she described being told to 'pull herself together'. She was sent to a psychologist who tried to state that she was school phobic and had an unhappy childhood. Eventually she had to resort to using a wheelchair, and after many visits to other doctors was finally diagnosed by Dr Speight. However as no local paediatrician accepted the diagnosis her problems were far from over. The conclusion drawn was that because her sister had diabetes she was pretending to be ill to gain attention. The family ultimately moved house to a new area. She was now well and attending University two years later than her peers.

What could be happening in the gut in ME?

Researchers in Belgium measured viral DNA in gastro-intestinal biopsies from 48 ME/CFS patients and 35 controls. Most viruses that were investigated were detected in a similar proportions in both groups with the exception of the parvovirus B19 which was found in 40% of ME/CFS patients and only 15% of the controls. This virus is linked, among others, to fifth disease (childhood disease of fever, malaise and skin rash), anaemia and a form of arthritis. The study suggests that at least in a subgroup of patients the parvovirus B19 may possibly be a cause of gastro-intestinal symptoms.

Researchers in Australia looked at lactic acid levels. D-lactic acidosis is a condition that arises from bacterial fermentation of carbohydrates in the gastro-intestinal tract leading to increased lactic acid levels in the blood. ME/CFS patients were found to have an increased lactic acid level. They also had an increase in streptococcus and enterococcus bacteria which could lead to heightened intestinal permeability (leaky gut) allowing lactic acid into the blood stream.

Klimas found that the intestinal barrier in the gut may be weakened by factors that are shown to trigger CFS such as psychological stress, physical stress such as strenuous exercise, allergies, surgery and trauma. These same factors can induce inflammation, activation of the immune system and oxidative stress (disturbances in the normal oxygen state of cells causing toxic effects). Inflammation may then cause 'leaky gut. Patients should be assessed for increased gut permeability and treated with anti-oxidants.

February 10th

It's a year since Chris has seen much more than the walls of his bedroom. He was feeling low and when Stu, a friend of Dougal's offered to take Chris to the cinema, it seemed sensible to try the outing. Chris said that he never seems to feel happy now. We prebooked the tickets and I then drove them to the Cinema. The drive took five minutes, and they only had about twenty yards to walk. This was followed by two days of exhaustion. "I did not think that going to the cinema could be so tiring!"

February 12th

We are still trying to get to the stage of the diet where Hayley [of the ME workshop] feels that we can start the anti-candida treatment. The swab we took indicates that Chris does have candida. He still cannot bring himself to drink only water. We have substituted squeezed lemon and fizzy water for all drinks, on Hayley's advice. I am impressed how seriously he is taking the diet, and he never breaks the rules.

What could be causing fatigue in ME?

Fatigue is an aspect of ME that is shared with other conditions such as cancer. Research in Antwerp shows that ME and cancer share abnormalities in the RNase L antiviral pathway and with a mechanism which regulates inflammation and oxidative stress. Natural Killer cell malfunction has been documented in both conditions. While there are clear differences between cancer and ME the researchers were intrigued by their shared abnormalities.

February 16th

Just when our spirits needed a lift, Danny provided it. Danny is Chris' closest friend. It is easy to like Danny; not only is he good looking, but he has an attractive personality and moreover he does not shy away from contact with adults. While I was opening the door to him today he told me that he had something for Chris. In his hand he had a large roll of white paper but I had no time to ask questions before the door of Chris' room was shut on the two of them.

Danny always has a mug of tea when he calls in, and I try and have some homemade biscuits ready as well, so I had an excuse to go back into the room. Danny was keen to show me what he had brought, and unrolled the paper.

"It's a scroll pledging that in 2004 when Chris and I leave school we are going round the world and we'll start by going to the Athens Olympics."

Only Danny, of all of us who know Chris, has the conviction that Chris will recover, and the courage to state it.

February 19th

On Chris' 16th birthday, in two months' time, he will have officially left school, and will no longer be eligible for Child Benefit. I decided to apply on his behalf for Incapacity Benefit. The Citizen's Advice Bureau have helped me to fill in the forms. I know that ME sufferers have huge problems in accessing benefits because the form does not lend itself to their type of disability, and I can now see why. If the disability isn't visible you don't 'fit'. It is not easy at his age to have to ask for money. If he was well he would probably be earning a bit and he would not have to ask.. Chris worries about the videos and games that I have bought him. I always say that the Child Benefit is for him and since he doesn't need shoes or clothes, he's entitled to be given what he does need, which are things to pass the time. Tomorrow Chris has to be seen by our GP.

February 20th

Chris never wants to see a doctor again and he was dreading the visit. I had asked Gran over because I thought if she was visiting he wouldn't think about it too much. As the time went on he went quieter and paler and finally went upstairs to his room. There is always this fear with ME sufferers that doctors won't believe their accounts of the illness. When our GP arrived I led the way upstairs to Chris' room where the curtains were closed. The doctor went and sat by Chris' bed and asked Chris to describe what he felt like. I prompted occasionally when Chris got tired, or lost for words. I could see that the doctor was interested and did believe what Chris was saying. "Do you ever feel down?" he asked. It is inevitable that people should think that they are just depressed. "Yes" said Chris "sometimes, but not for long." Chris' face was a dirty white colour and his eyelids heavy and puffed. ME sufferers economise on expressive movements and never make unnecessary gesticulations or modulate their voices as we are accustomed to do. At the end of the interview the doctor, before he stood up to leave, said, "Chris, I can see this is not a nice illness and there is little that I can do to help, but if there is anything that I can do, I will."

We went downstairs and I thanked the doctor for coming. "What a remarkably mature young man Chris is," he remarked as he stopped by the door, "and what a horrendous disease."

February 27th

"This is the first time I have felt happy". Diet is almost sugar free. Chris is doing more on the computer, not sure what, probably games.

February 28th

From whatever angle you look at it, Christmas, as it used to be, did not work. It only emphasised how things have changed. Alex had said in exasperation when it was over, "Next Christmas we are going to the States." I have now booked the tickets. We all need something to look forward to, and if the worst happened, which I can hardly bear to think about, and we were unable to go because Chris was still this ill, then we would have to cancel. If we don't book now to visit Iain and Becca we will never get tickets nearer the time.

March 7th

Chris has had a horrid week when he was unable to control his pattern of short nights and disturbed sleep. He tried twice walking the twenty yards to the post-box. However yesterday was his 'Best day yet'. Chris started a scrapbook and juggling. He is managing to watch more taxing films and to write bits of film scripts on the computer.

He has also been in the kitchen to heat up food a couple of times. The first time he came through to the kitchen and offered to slice an onion for me, I was as alarmed as if he had asked if he could train for a half marathon and I had to check myself for being so fearful. He seems to be allergic to carrots; he hates them, saying that they give him twitchy legs. Frozen peas also seem to cause his legs to twitch. I've noticed that a low mood can be rectified by food, and that is what Iain picked up on years ago. Apart from a small amount of chocolate each day, Chris is virtually on the dairy, wheat and sugar free diet that he needs to be on before we can introduce the anti-candida pills.

Are there links between Glandular Fever and ME?

Glandular Fever, also known as Infectious Mononucleosis or 'Mono' in USA, or Epstein Barr virus or the kissing disease, is characterised by fever, sore throat and fatigue. As many as 12% of adults can go on to develop ME after contracting Glandular Fever. A survey of 301 adolescents in Chicago discovered that the figure was 13%. Of this group 7% were still ill at 12 months and 4% after 2 years.

March 9th

Danny and Angela called in and Stu spent the night in the flat while I went down to Galloway to treat my patients.

March 16th

No more chocolate! The only substitute available is orange or raspberry flavoured carob bars which are only bearable because there is no alternative. Dougal's reaction to them is an indication of how desperate you have to be to eat them. He says that eating them is the equivalent of eating dog food. Hayley, who is the telephone contact for the ME Network, says we can now start the anti-candida treatment. Hayley's sister is the nutritionist whose expertise helped Caroline Brownbill to recover. Once Chris starts the diet he has to stick to it rigidly.

March 17th

Chris has started taking one tablet of mycopryl a day. Mycopryl is found in coconuts and it prevents the coconut milk from going off. Mycopryl attacks the candida which now has nothing to feed on because it is being starved of sugar. If there is no reaction after a week, he will increase to two tablets. If there is a reaction you wait until it settles before increasing the dose.

March 24th

"These pills have really mucked up my dreams, everything I was ever scared of has come back." Chris is feeling sick and in desperation I went to HMV and bought him the next series of "Friends". My antidote to his miserable moments.

After he had had another poor night Hayley suggested that Chris changed the time that he took the pills from 6 pm to 11 am. She explained that the mycopryl is working by killing off the candida and as the toxins leave the body the ME symptoms return very strongly. She called this 'die off'. She urged him not to give up. It is impossible not to be heartened by her sympathetic, lilting, Welsh voice.

March 30th

We all moved to Galloway for the Easter break. It has not been too bad a weekend. Chris is feeling easier and has had the odd two minute walk around the garden. Hayley was right, now the toxins have cleared he does seem better.

April 4th

What a long time it has been before we could hear these words. "I'm feeling better". Since he started taking the pills Chris has been cold and tired and has stayed upstairs in bed, feeling lethargic. He has been waking at 1 or 2 pm, but not even watching videos. Now he is playing computer games and trying to read 'Fight Club' script. He finds board games difficult but is playing a bit of snooker.

April 9th

Chris has had a week with no reaction to the mycopril and he increasing to two a day. Katie and Dougal came for the weekend. What a welcome relief! I can hand over some of my entertaining duties! Chris is needing a change from me and he is so happy. He is not having as many sweating spells.

April 10th

Very happy, sunny spell. Sleep 2 am-11.20 am today.

April 12th

There seems to be no reaction to 2 pills a day so today we will increase the dose to 3 pills. Chris drinks fizzy water with lemon. He drinks loads of water, especially in the morning when he tends to feel at his worst.. Alex went to the Supermarket and bought a bottle of gin, 2 tonics, 8 large bottles of carbonated water and 20 lemons.

April 21st

Reasonably steady spell. Sleeping longer. "I now think I can say to people that I am getting better."

April 22nd

Chris' 16th birthday. Ask any mother with a child who has this condition and they will tell you the huge sense of relief that they feel when their child turns sixteen. Chris is no longer required to go to school. We are no longer at risk of being scrutinised by any local authority or social services personnel. The cases coming to light, documented by Panorama, of children being taken from their families or having their cases examined by a school Reporter because they are not at school, are alarming. It is a scenario that every family with a child with ME fears. There are cases of very sick children being removed from their families and locked in secure psychiatric units. Dr Speight said "psychiatrists are diagnosing mothers as having Münchausen[-syndrome]-by-Proxy and there is enormous pressure on sick children to attend school with mandatory involvement by paediatric psychiatrists."

> What are the NICE guidelines?
>
> National Institute for Health and Clinical Excellence is an independent organisation responsible for giving national guidance on the promotion of good health and the treatment and prevention of ill health.
> It is intended for use by clinicians.
> The NICE guidelines for CFS are:- maintaining and if possible extending your emotional and physical abilities: Managing the physical and emotional effects of your symptoms.
> Suggested management strategies. CBT: GET: Activity management: Medication for pain relief: Antidepressants for sleep.

April 23rd

My birthday. We spent it back in Edinburgh putting up the posters we had given Chris for his birthday. All film-related of course. Tarantino, Pulp Fiction, Apocalypse Now, Small Time Crooks, and one of Bart Simpson. I went up the ladder while Chris directed proceedings. I had painted his room blue with an orange alcove last autumn and hung curtains with shades of orange, yellow and red. Since the curtains are permanently drawn, it gives the illusion of light, and I understand that blue is a healing colour. It is what he chose anyway.

April 28th

Chris had no sleep last night and had a very shaky day. Recently he's been getting to sleep at 5 am. We tried backgammon. It would be nice to have a change from cards which we have played now for about a year. The strict diet continues, lemon and water, sausages and bacon for breakfast, ham and salad for 'lunch' at around 4 pm, crisps for snack and for supper, mince, onions and peppers with potatoes and broccoli. He is still on 3 mycopril and is having sweats but no other horrid symptoms at present.

Then he surprised me. "Mum, I know you will say no, but I think I'd like to learn some French."

May 5th

Chris is on to four pills. He says his sleep is weird but that he is feeling better. He wrote a few thank you cards. And went to the cinema with Andy.

Chris slept for nine hours after he'd been to the cinema, but he dreams all night and was tired until after midday.

May 6th

Best day for ages. Started ten minutes of French. Probably the best he's been since the day of the newspaper article.

May 7th

Two good nights. "Do you know why I have been sleeping better? It's because my head is not so hot. It's different from having the fan on."

We notice that the spots on Chris' face clear up when he feels better, sometimes almost from one minute to the next, although they can reappear just as suddenly. He used to have a lot of mouth sores even as a young child and these too came and went spontaneously. The nursery doctor ticked me off for giving him too many lollies.

May 10th

Chris feels dizzy. I notice that his face looks more swollen. When he was in bed last year his skin looked waterlogged and puffy and he lost all the contours of his face around his jaw and ears. This has come back again, perhaps due to the increase in pills or perhaps because he is doing more mental work. That is, if ten minutes of French can be considered too much work.

May 13th

Five pills have really done it. All the ME symptoms are back. He's been especially bad from midday yesterday until 4pm today. His curtains are closed. He can only watch television. He's not hungry and everything tastes funny. He is sweating, pale and yet feels cold, and is sitting with his feet up.

Hayley says "Hold on in there. This is the body getting rid of toxins." But it has taken five days so far.

May 24th

Friends called in after their exams. It has been a lonely time for Chris with everyone on exam leave. Now that the exams are under way they may call in more often as they head home at odd times of the day.

He had his worst night for ages. I ended up chatting with him at 3 am again. I have got into the habit, if I wake in the night, of going along the passage to see if Chris is still awake. I tuck up under his downy at the foot of his bed and sit with it around my shoulders and listen as he tells me his latest views regarding the direction or lighting or whatever of the films he has been watching. This time all his left side was twitchy and he was needing to have company until it settled down. Hayley advises that we stop the pills for a few days.

June 6th
Becca and Iain are here for the mid term week. Chris had two nights of short spells of sleep and one spell when he was awake for twenty four hours. Then suddenly he slept from 7pm to 7am. "Congratulations, Chris!"

"I'm being congratulated for something over which I have no control whatever!" He commented, appreciating the irony. He is still sweating but is cheerful. He is not eating much but has restarted the pills. Danny has been to stay. And then Dougal joined us for three days. The weather is good and they have a diabolo craze. I found Chris in tears yesterday evening. He had had a good day and thought that he was, on the whole, better, but it had not lasted.

June 30th
Chris has had one week of 7 mycropryl tablets with no reaction. Now we can stop. It has taken about three months altogether to complete the treatment. It is difficult to know where to go from here. Hayley said that a systemic toxin remover, like oregano, might be the next stage.

I have heard from one of his past teachers that one of Chris' old school friends has got ME. He struggled through standard grades but now has dropped out of school and is very depressed. Apparently his friend had become very unpopular and had said at one time that he always hurt the people he least wanted to.

July 1st
Neal came to stay and he and Chris got very excited about the Henman Match. But now that he has gone the summer stretches ahead more bleakly than last year. This time we know how long the holidays feel, and how lonely they are. People ask you what you are doing this summer and you pause with a mixture of embarrassment and apology before answering.

I once asked my former superintendent the same question and she told me falteringly that they did not take holidays because their son had depression. I now understood how awkward she felt. Sometimes I explain and sometimes I just say that we are taking a Christmas break.

Subjects for conversation are so limited that when Alex and I do go out I invariably find myself talking about ME and hating myself at the same time for boring the other person. It is difficult to explain how every waking moment - and there are plenty at night too - is spent thinking how you can help your child get better. If you are out you feel guilty. You just know that they need you all the time. As one mother said to me in a letter, "How quickly would she sink if I was not there?"

> What happens to muscles in ME?
>
> One study examined what happened in the calf muscles of ME patients during exercise and compared them to controls. The ME patient's 'proton efflux' which is a measure of how their muscles handle acid was reduced immediately after exercise. It also took them longer to reach maximum, and this maximum was lower than the maximum proton efflux of the controls. This signifies an impairment of the proton excretion in the recovery phase following exercise; ie ME patients recover from exercise substantially more slowly than healthy controls. Researchers think it is likely that autonomic nervous system abnormalities may be responsible as the results in the muscles would be post-exertional symptoms of fatigue. The researchers, in Newcastle, are now looking at the function of a possible under performing energy-generating enzyme in ME patients.

July 7th

The oregano pills are causing more tiredness.

I rang Liz this morning. She is a particularly understanding friend who lives about half-an-hour's drive away, to ask if we could go over occasionally to enable Chris to play snooker on their full-sized table for a change. Then I burst into tears. Not helpful really.

I have been reading some of my father-in-law's old papers and it struck me that I have got to stop worrying. That I have to trust that Chris is going to get better because nothing that I do can make it happen. In fact if stress makes it worse, and Chris senses that I am worrying, it could be counter-productive. You could go round in circles with this illness.

I told my cousin Caroline, when I saw her yesterday, that Chris was finally starting to improve and she said "Well done!" Not at all what I was expecting but still very nice.

July 9th

I have been having the weirdest and most vivid dreams. I'm in a home, the upstairs and downstairs are connected by a ladder that might be used to access an attic but there is no ground floor in between the two. There are a lot of very busy staff but they are not interested in us. There is gross overcrowding. My bed is lower and narrower than everyone else's and the mattress does not fit because it is too short. There is a full size bed next to mine. It is Chris' but his mattress is only a foot wide and shaped like a canoe. All of us are wobbly with different balance problems and varying degrees of in-coordination. I am one of the least affected and I am allowed to go from room to room. The upstairs room is more spacious and full of specially designed wooden toys like clever swings, but one of the staff tells me we are not supposed to have any fun.

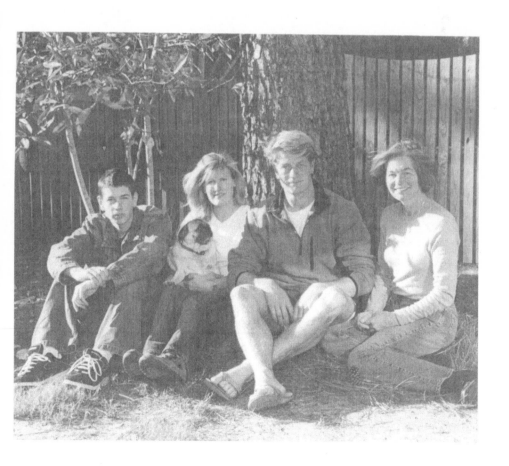

2002 Summer

"No blessed leisure for love or hope
But only time for grief!"

Thomas Hood

When the Child Benefit form came through stating that payments would come to a halt after Chris' sixteenth birthday unless he continued in full-time education, I had decided to explore what money he might be entitled to. This was more an angry reaction to the fact that he could not, rather than would not, attend school. Chris had always been distressed when I had bought him things, he had, even at thirteen, been able to earn his pocket money by doing jobs for us. I wanted him to feel independent financially especially as he had to rely on me for every other aspect of his life.

Without Benefits from the state some ME patients could not survive. Many live in extremely straightened circumstances, not having the stamina to persist with applications or to lodge an appeal. Some are so sick that they do not claim anything at all and are totally reliant on their families. Two such sufferers are aged twenty-five and twenty-eight. On entering secondary school, both were highly intelligent and actively sporty. Neither are in a wheelchair. Why are they unable to access benefits? One reason is that the process is so arduous that they have neither the physical nor mental stamina to undergo the form filling followed by the physical examination. The second reason is that they can go up stairs, pick something off the floor, heat through a meal or walk from the car to have their hair cut. All these are the sort of questions demanded by the disability forms. What these two can not do is repeat these actions, or be able to do them when they need to. Even more disabling to both, though unquantifiable, is their brain fatigue. If they were to obtain work what use is their ten minute attention span to an employer? Finally, should either of these two young people complete the process, who can guarantee that they will not be ill for days, if not weeks from the effort involved? After all, both of them were subjected as young teenagers to coercion in complying with either an exercise regime or school attendance. This left them more sick than they had been prior to these activities, and from which they have never recovered.

> **Why is it difficult to access Benefits?**
>
> To access benefits patients have to undergo assessments. These assessments are primarily designed for those people with physical disabilities. In some cases ME patients are assessed as having a mental illness which reduces the amount to which a person is entitled. Patients with private insurance are equally as likely to struggle to receive an adequate pay out. ME is not recognised as a medical label and the applicant is reliant on the judgement of the assessor.

July 14th
"Do you ever think, 'why me?'" Jeremy asked. "Never!" Chris replied simply.

July 16th
"I have no idea what part of the year we are in, it's all a blur."

July 17th
The Disability Doctor came this afternoon to assess Chris. The doctor, a quiet, reserved man, arrived holding a wad of papers on a clipboard and I led the way upstairs to Chris' room. Chris had shrunk into himself. If the doctor decided against an allowance it would confirm for Chris that the world in general did not believe he was ill.

"What do you have to do for Chris that you did not have to do for your other two boys at his age?" This single question put the whole interview in context. I relaxed. Of course what I do for Chris is probably more than I would have to do even for a five-year-old, because it includes broken nights and the fact that for most of the time I am his only company.

As he left I asked the doctor if he knew of any other cases, if he had any ideas on treatment? He was guarded. He was only there to assess.

July 20th
Meanwhile the BMJ have listed 174 conditions that it considers are not diseases. ME finds itself right in the centre of the list along with such conditions as aging, boredom, freckles and big ears. *The Guardian* comments that the BMJ list is set to affront some groups.

July 24th

It becomes an obsession, this sleep problem. It is almost as if Chris will get better the minute he can sleep. Last night he slept from 2 am-10 am but was very restless. At the moment he says that food is tasteless and that he has a stiff neck. Chris has a septic toe and eczema but is wearing shoes, the curtains are open and he is able to read. He had a good spell from 6-8 pm this evening and started planning a book based on the Mafia. I find that none of Chris' plans really last, like the Maths that lasted a couple of days, or the French which lasted a bit longer, before his brain closes down again. You always hope that this time it won't.

July 28th

He has had two 'scary nights', as he calls them. He has finished taking the oregano, and we have seen no further improvement. We went on to 'Putrid and Rancid', Jane's name for the supplements that Chris was taking to try to help his adrenal function, but have stopped them after talking to Hayley. She suggested that he probably needs a break from treatment. Instead, I made some yeast-free bread because he is still sticking to the diet. It was declared delicious, but an upset stomach followed.

I bought some new shoes 'on spec' and discovered that Chris has gone up two sizes. His toe seems to be a bit better and I wonder whether it was because his shoes were so small that the nail became infected. However, he has hardly been wearing shoes often enough to cause an injury. He is probably just going rotten!

August 6th

Chris has spent two nights with Helen and her family which has broken up this tedious spell.

Also four friends from his old school called in for forty minutes because they were doing some sailing in the area. What a boost for Chris!

August 7th

Chris was better immediately without the most recent homeopathic pills. They must have been too strong for him. Alex and I are going away for two nights and Chris is going to stay with Jean and Jimmy.

August 10th

To my relief there was no adverse reaction to the visit to Jean and Jimmy and now Dougal and Katie are staying. Chris came with me to meet them from Prestwick Airport, which was a good surprise for them. Chris has made an Airfix model, and has spent some time outside.

August 20th

I really wonder if I am getting ME or MS or something because my leg muscles are twitching when I am in bed. This happened once before, when Helen's mother was diagnosed with her brain tumour and I could not sleep. If anyone talks too long when they come to see me, my head just buzzes. My co-ordination is awful and if I am pruning in the garden I am convinced that I am going to cut off the fingers of my left hand. It is probably just having broken nights for over eighteen months, but it makes me wonder what on earth would happen if I got ill as well. There are families where the mother, too, has developed ME. There is no evidence to prove that ME is contagious, except that all early accounts reported were of epidemics, yet there are a disproportionate amount of families where there are siblings with ME.

August 21st

Chris has been to stay overnight with Ian H and managed well. "Isn't it exciting? It's odd because although I feel okay all day I still know there are things I can't do." He had a few drives at the driving range one day, and ten minutes hitting tennis balls on another.

August 24th

I was sitting sewing this afternoon when Chris came down the stairs wearing a t-shirt and pyjama bottoms, and his shoes. He has not been feeling great since returning from Ian's and he had been particularly grumpy in the morning. "If I just act normal then I'll be normal," he stated as he walked past me and out of the front door. I watched him cross the yard, go into the shed and emerge pushing his mountain bike. We had bought the bike for his thirteenth birthday but even in that year he had hardly ridden it. I stood, horrified, as he did two circuits round the yard. He started a third and then dropped the bike onto the ground. He came back into the house, dragged his legs up the stairs and slammed his bedroom door. I left him for a while. When I went into his room he had the Play Station control in his hands and did not take his eyes off the screen.

His statement is a reasonable one. When you are well, making yourself do something can lift you out of the doldrums. But not when you are ill.

September 3rd

School has restarted and his new form teacher called in for a chat with Chris just to keep him in touch. It is exceptionally good of her to do that since he is not registered at the school.

September 5th

This weekend Neal spent the night and they went to the cinema. Unfortunately Chris' ability to fall asleep is slipping to 3 am.

September 7th

There are no closed curtains, gloves or thick socks at the moment. Chris' colour is better and he only puts his feet up in the evening. He is excited at the prospect of seeing his school friends again. He is tired but not feeling awful. He did his first short walk to the nearest lamp post for quite a while. "I know I can walk to the bus stop, but I know I can't get to Princes Street even if they say it's mind over matter." he told me. I have noticed that he is on his feet for longer lengths of time.

> Why is the label Münchausen syndrome by proxy feared by ME families?
>
> Münchausen syndrome by proxy (MSBP) is an uncommon psychiatric condition. Typically a child is reported ill by their main carer, usually the mother, who exaggerates or fabricates illness in the child. It is thought that the perpetrator feels satisfaction by gaining the attention and sympathy of doctors and nurses. No symptoms are found in the child.
> Because regular tests in ME children prove negative, and because the patient is a child, the criteria for diagnosing MSBP can be considered by some professionals. The rate of diagnosis of MSBP in ME children is four times the rate than that found in the general population. The treatment for MSBP is to remove the child from its parents.

September 12th

We took a taxi to HMV. Imagine what a taxi driver must think when asked to drive a perfectly fit-looking teenager and his obviously able mother to a shop no more than seven minutes walk away! I was very aware of this and felt some explanation was called for, but on the other hand I did not want to embarrass Chris. I opted for the first course of action and I think that Chris was happy about it, since I did not get the typical teenager's exasperated warning of 'Mum', and the taxi driver took us as close to the shop as he could.

Once he had chosen his DVDs, Chris left the purchasing up to me. I think this was in case he was asked anything by the cashier because he can't cope with instant decisions.

We caught a bus from outside the shop. The walk from the bus stop to the flat, a quick three minutes walk for me, was, through Chris' eyes, quite a hike.

September 16th

Chris went on to have three poor days He has been feeling sick in the morning but has managed to play scrabble with me and to do a bit of French. He went to the lamp post and back but says that he is tired, which is not surprising since he has been unable to sleep until 4 am. He is looking forward to Danny coming to stay at the weekend and they plan, with my help as chauffeur, to go to the cinema.

September 18th

Perhaps he has been attempting too much but, whether he has or not, today has been the biggest disaster since he first fell ill.

Chris cannot get to a barber, and attempts at cutting his hair with scissors were so bad that we took Danny's advice and bought our own trimmers. Alex usually cuts Chris' hair for him with two blades, one 7mm and one 3mm, I think. Today Chris did his own and came into the kitchen to show me, running his hand along the top of his head. "This bit does not feel quite right," he said and picking up the trimmer went back to the mirror.

The comb had fallen off leaving the blade exposed and Chris did one long shave from the front to the back of his scalp. His scalp was bisected by a wide groove slightly off to the left of centre. I could not conceal my alarm when Chris returned to the kitchen. He took one look at my face, went to look at himself in the hall mirror and then sliding down the wall cradled his head in his hands and sank onto his heels. There was nothing I could do except to await his reaction.

"This is just one more thing to keep me shut in," he said bitterly and was unable to control his tears.

September 21st

Chris was soon able to laugh at himself and his haircut, and Dougal and Katie convinced him that it was the very latest style in fashion. It may be, but it is permanently hidden under the beanie hat that he sent me out to buy.

Chris' school friends were in again yesterday, the four of them barely miss a Thursday. They suggested that Chris might like to go to the school concert on Monday. I said I would drop him off and pick him up. He is excited but nervous. He says he feels detached and dissociated from everything. "I don't know how to be my age."

September 24th

It's the September break. I am trying to plan something for Chris for October, because he will have no visits that fortnight. It is a question of balancing the risks with the benefits, and also how to prevent any of his friends who might be prepared to spend time with him from being bored when physical activity has to be avoided. Henny has suggested that he might like to go and stay with her. She suggested that he could use a golf buggy to go through the grounds of the hotel to play snooker.

While there is the slightest risk of there being damage to Chris by exercise, I shall go on being cautious. The other mothers that I am in contact with are equally as cautious, and some of them have learnt the hard way because their children were put through graded exercise. Davina is still as poorly as ever with severe cognitive problems. Alice's son, who failed to improve while on the programme, was told that he was not trying hard enough. He had been severely ill with dysphasia (unable to speak) and confusion when at his worst, but he is beginning to recover and planning to do his Highers at a technical college.

September 28th

Chris has come back from Galloway with Alex's guitar and is trying out a few chords. He is not playing so many Play Station games now, and his choice of films is becoming more erudite. Until recently the ones he chose were all action, or violent eighteen-rated films. Now, when I go with my list to HMV, I notice that there are more fifteens among them and that he has chosen films with more substance to them. He says that he can never see a film in one session because he can not concentrate, which is why action films are so much easier. I have stopped being embarrassed when taking my lists into HMV or to Electronic Boutique, especially the latter, where I join the queue of youngsters, all of us clutching our exchanges.

September 30th

If Chris does go to Henny's for the October break he is going to need some clothes. He has been onto the NEXT website and has chosen some

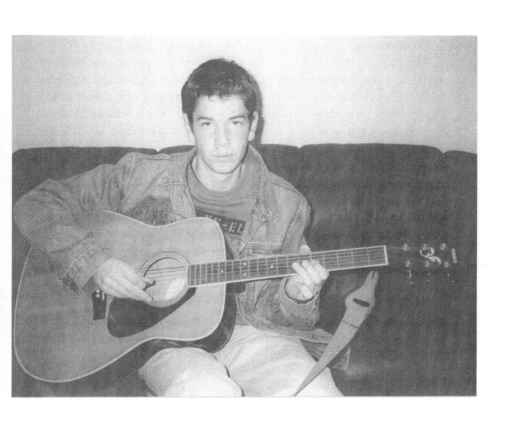

for me to buy. The faithful Danny is going to spend part of the break with Chris. It is giving him something to look forward to.

October 1st
Henny confirmed that Chris and Danny can stay with her during the October break. It is a three hour drive from Edinburgh so we will see how he survives this jaunt.

October 2nd
Chris is still sticking to the diet and it does not seem to be much of an effort. I gave up chocolate to keep him company and we agree that we neither of us bother about it any more. Chris actually says that it makes him feel sick. Nor does he miss sweets or sugar. I've warned him about Aspartame, often used as a sugar substitute, which has a much more potent effect on the brain than sugar. Sugar gives the body a 'high' and the person feels a surge of energy. There is always a corresponding 'low', rather like a diabetic 'hypo' where the person feels horrid. It is this low that the sugar-avoidance diet tries to prevent. On the whole we do not talk about ME, nor do I ask how he is because I soon learnt to read the signs. He is interesting to talk to, with few of the impenetrable teenage patches that you might expect. I have learnt when to suggest a game of cards, or when just to sit beside him and do my tapestry, when to suggest that I go and rent a video or stay and make him a meal. I have to be ready to forego a task, or delay going to bed if he asks, because he only does so when he really needs it. He remains considerate of the implications of his illness on our lives, even reminding me one day that I had not been for my walk.

October 9th
Chris is wearing thinner socks but his toe is still a nuisance. His feet do not go such a horrid blue colour when he puts his feet to the floor. His hands get cold when he plays the guitar, but so far the craze continues. He finished the Teach Yourself the Guitar book that I got him in one week and has asked for 'The Strokes'— the American rock band — tabs. He watches guitarists on his videos and learns from them.

October 30th
Chris said very little about his week away. Danny stayed for three days and those were obviously very happy. After that, despite Henny's considerateness, he was lonely, and weary from the unaccustomed

company. Henny is very understanding with Chris and she has given Alex and me an opportunity to recharge our batteries. I am aware that many mothers are not so fortunate.

November 7th
Chris' weekly outing seems to be coming to the supermarket with me. He prowls around the shopping aisles like a sightseer. He has found that he can not walk every day and so we have stopped setting any targets. However he has been for his first walk at night. "I find that I'm not frightened in the streets at night, but I'm not sure about Galloway because of the burglary. Henny says it's because I can't put a face to the men." I am sure she's right. What is in your head is often more frightening than reality. I'm also sure that when his head recovers from the ME that he will find that all these fears will resolve. He had been fine going around Edinburgh and meeting up with friends when he had first arrived. It had only been latterly, as he started to show signs of lack of stamina, that he had begun to be reluctant to do so. It alarmed me too that he found the streets overwhelming where previously he had relished the freedom.

November 10th
Thank heavens for the guitar, as reading is impossible again. Chris' fingers are raw but he is able to play for 3 or 4 hours in the day. He is studying every frame of the 'Strokes' video to decide what sort of clothes are being worn and he has sent Dougal and me on shopping searches for him.

November 11th
Chris has been a bit low, because his year are all studying hard and have not been in touch.
However Danny called in today with an entry form for a short film competition which his English teacher, Mr Hart, had given to him. Mr Hart had said that if they are interested he would be prepared to help them. This has given Chris a great boost, and plenty of food for thought..

November 12th
Chris always makes allowances for his friends if they do not call in. He knows that it must be boring for them. It's boring enough for him! He may get low but he has not been depressed. It is possible to tell the difference. There are complicated charts which show how sleeping patterns vary, early waking for depression and late waking for ME,

What can we learn from over-training syndrome?
High Intensity Exercise. Papers from the First Rugby World Cup Conference 1991

The immune system's function is to protect the body from harmful micro-organisms. By studying athletes at the highest level of their sport who succumb to overtraining with its accompanying susceptibility to infections we can learn what is happening in the very earliest stages of ME/CFS. The symptoms are similar. All athletes can suffer from tiredness, depression and sleep disturbances, but what they notice is underperformance. This is noticed at the very outset. This is unlike the situation that an average person who has a lower optimum threshold would meet. The latter can continue to function for very much longer before underperformance (at work or school for example) is apparent.

Several mechanisms are involved and muscles feature prominently. Muscles are a source of fuel for the immune system, if they are injured then the immune system is compromised. If they are overused there are remarkable similarities between their response to exercise and that seen in an inflammatory response to infection. Thus to exercise while fighting a virus would increase the detrimental effect on the athlete. Treatments to suppress infection give the athletes the appearance of being fit and well and being able to train, but when they compete it is obvious that they are not fit. Because athletes' blood is tested very early once they contract a virus many abnormalities show up in their blood.

When a person with ME/CFS presents with problems they are at a very much lower level of health before loss of performance is evident. Exercise would compound the assault on their body, as with an athlete. Unfortunately the delay in testing means that any virus that might have shown up initially is unlikely to be detected.

Tests on athletes showed that recruitment of muscles is compromised since both the brain and the muscles compete for the same amino acids. A decrease in levels in the brain may contribute to the decrease in maximal work capacity by the muscles. In ME/CFS this might explain the extra effort that these people have to make in order to achieve their usual muscle activity and their reported perception of increased effort.

Furthermore, on the treadmill, there was seen to be no loss of motivation in ME/CFS patients. Nor was there any evidence of increased levels of end-tidal CO_2 which means that their reduced output was not due to over breathing. (This should be kept in mind when considering McEvedy's theory of hysteria).

The important lesson that can be drawn from these papers, and which is one explanation for curbing exercise, is their mode of management. Even with a slight fall in performance levels athletes are completely rested for 3-6 weeks. Return to training is slowly introduced over three months or they found that the athlete would relapse.

exercise is tolerated by those with depression as is alcohol, both of which make ME patients worse. However it is the lack of motivation that distinguishes depression from ME. I think of him as 'being down' rather than being depressed. ME is often treated by the same methods that are used for depression but one mother told me that when her ME daughter was clinically depressed for about four months and she asked for help she couldn't get it. Yet, as she pointed out, doctors are quick enough to treat these children as having depression.

November 19th

It's inconceivable that we have done nothing for two years, and yet this is what this illness demands. The loss of normal brain function that ME sufferers experience is the cruellest aspect of this illness. It is the part that is hidden to the casual observer and which is so distressing to those who are in regular contact and who try to help. When you consider the effect that ME has on their brains all other features of the illness take second place. The lack of exercise, fresh air and light, social contact and family gatherings, parties, and holidays which are all modified or disappear, would be bearable, if they had control of their brain function.

My coping strategy is always to have something in the pipeline even if it has to be cancelled, and so I have decided to take Chris on the train to my sister's for three days. No walking is involved except from the taxi to the train and once we are there he will have a new set of videos and a change of scene. My sister and brother-in-law have thought out various ways of helping that have touched me. Firstly they invited Alex and me to join them on holiday in Corsica. Secondly they have arranged a monthly subscription to a film magazine for Chris' last birthday. It is so nice to have post when you are confined to base, and magazines are perfect for scrambled brains.

Now they are meeting us off the train and delivering us back again. David has invited me down to London before, and suggested that I just leave Chris with a child-minder. It was hard to explain how very much more difficult it is to leave a teenager with a carer than it would be to leave a younger child who is used to being looked after. I felt as if I was making excuses not to go, and I was, because I am so protective about who Chris is left with. The demands of the job are unique and paramount is the ability of the person not to over stimulate him. This trip will give me some idea if our planned visit to USA next month is viable. It will help me to gauge if the journey would be a foolish risk to his slowly improving health.

November 25th

Chris was easily upset today. He was exhausted from composing and writing the film script with Danny. They only had to write the synopsis but the wording had to be precise. The work took about an hour which is an extremely long concentration span for him. Their story line is about a man who finds a card in his pocket inviting him to a meeting. When he follows up the appointment he finds himself mixing with a terrorist organisation. He is then unable to extricate himself and there is inevitably a tragic ending.

November 28th

I dropped Chris at school to meet with Danny and Mr Hart who is going over the synopsis with them. Chris was elated when I picked him up. Mr Hart has offered to tutor him in English. He will go in once before the end of term to discuss what form it should take. Since Chris finds reading an effort he suggested that essay writing might be a start.

This morning Chris announced. "I dreamt that Dougal, Iain, Dad and I were all in a breakfast place and that I had everyone in the place in stitches."

December 3rd

Over Christmas Chris and I will spend a month with Iain and Becca to make the effort worth while and Alex will join us for ten days. I am puzzled why Chris is indifferent about going. I am not allowing myself to contemplate the possibility that he might not be well enough to travel and perhaps he too is aware of this. His condition has been relatively stable for some time and minor excursions have only left him with a mild exacerbation of symptoms and I am cautiously hopeful.

December 6th

Chris waited all day, becoming more and more miserable, for Danny to arrive as planned. Finally at 4 pm he persuaded himself that he was being unreasonable and settled down to his guitar and cheered up.

December 7th

Danny and his younger brother came for two hours today.

December 11th

"I find it fascinating that Chris can't cope with decisions." Alex observed when we were discussing whether we should take Chris to a doctor about his septic toe. To defend Chris I jumped down poor Alex's throat, although this was not justified because I had observed exactly the same trait. I have tried since July to allow him to make up his own mind regarding his daily life. When he is very unwell, however, he is like a diabetic who is having a 'hypo' incident, and he finds it impossible to think rationally.

December 12th
Last night Chris rattled off a short story. It consisted of four pages and included seven characters.

Not a wonder he is brain dead and could not think when playing scrabble with Alex and me in the evening. We are keeping a tally of the amount of times each of us wins. His present run is twenty-one to my nine. Alex does not play often enough to qualify.

December 15th
Lots of Chris' friends called in before we left for the States which was a great send-off. What is more, I slept through, or failed to set, my alarm and it was only thanks to Chris that we set off in time for the flight. I had been worrying not only about how far we would have to walk but also whether there would be suitable food for him on the flight. Altogether I had become a totally anxious Mother, and had taken ages to fall asleep.

In fact the journey was relatively easy and uneventful.

December 19th
The first two days have been relaxed and easy. Becca is between jobs and Iain's work goes slack around now. Today Chris is 'paying' for the journey and feels very rough. I, on the other hand, have slept for twelve hours every night. I feel quite different here. I have shed a great load of responsibility because no longer do I have to be Chris' sole companion. All I have to do while I am here is to look after his health by providing the right foods and watching that he paces himself. I notice that he is taking the latter seriously and I rarely have to intervene which makes the balance between us so much easier.

December 20th
Alex arrived today. The weather has been good and sunny but Chris' face has reacted. The skin is red and raw and if he smiles the skin cracks. We ended up by going to one of the twenty-four hour clinics and, for £72, we were given a tube of steroid cream! The amount did include the consultation.

December 27th

Chris had half a glass of champagne at our meal on Christmas day and then had a poor day. He himself thought it was the drink. A friend of Iain's has lent Chris his guitar.

December 28th

Iain has planned a road trip so that we can have a holiday without exerting Chris. He has hired a People Carrier for us, and we are going to drive along the Outer Banks.

2003

"There is no past, present or future.
Using tenses to divide time is like making chalk marks on water."

Janet Frame

This could be called the year of convalescence, although it was not apparent in the early months as Chris 'paid' for pushing out the boundaries while in USA. After two or three months his condition settled down and recovery was noticeable. It all happened so slowly, and there were such variables from day to day, and from parts of one day. Weeks would tick by without my being conscious of whether Chris was making progress or merely marking time. Convalescence is a word hardly used in medicine nowadays, but it is one that is familiar to a generation who nursed childhood illnesses without the benefit of vaccinations or antibiotics.

I did wonder if I had not sent Chris back to school immediately he was better after each of his bouts of illness whether he would have recovered more completely and never ultimately succumbed to full blown ME. Neither Chris, nor I, wanted him to miss any more school than was necessary. Moreover it is now incumbent on a parent, if the child is off school for more than three days, to produce a doctor's sick note. Few parents want to bother a doctor for a note when, hopefully, by the third day the child is already recovering.

The arrival of anti-inflammatory drugs, aspirin for lowering temperatures, and anti-biotics for tacking bacterial infections has meant that people are no longer ill as they used to be in the old fashioned sense. Early return to school is therefore possible but essentially the child is still 'under the weather'. Could the huge increase in post-viral fatigue syndromes and chronic fatigue states be caused by ignoring the body's need to convalesce?. It would be interesting to discover, in the light of the observations that in outbreaks of ME it was the active staff and not the recumbent patients who contracted the illness, whether active schoolchildren are more likely to suffer from CFS syndromes. Whatever the outcome of that particular discussion, I had decided that in Chris' case we would exercise extreme caution, and follow Dr Speight's advice of patience and avoiding undue exertion. I am certain that it contributed to his ultimate recovery.

January 1st

The road trip. Chris' first taste of real life. He can now manage a good session of activity each day but needs the liberty to opt out at any time. I am encouraged how he can pace himself and judge his capabilities. After the morning at Jockey's Ridge, which is a huge sandbank, both he and Iain were stiff though Iain was doing somersaults where Chris just went to the top to watch. Walking along the boardwalk in Washington the following day we had only gone seven minutes when Chris asked if we had to go so fast. Iain opted to walk back to the Chevy Astro with him.

January 4th

Chris' feet are still a problem with poor circulation and poisoned toe, his "gross toe", as it seems to be called, but his face has cleared up with the medication the doctor gave him and in fact he looks better than he has done for ages. Before the skin reaction his spots were awful and now they have all have vanished. I had forgotten to get some micro-chips today, or to do some potatoes, and the corn tortillas are horrid, so Chris is low on food. My fault. He does not say anything but goes pale and quiet.

January 6th

Becca was quite excited that she and Iain had been able to arrange some contact for Chris with people of his own age. Chris, on the other hand was not so sure. Brittany, one of the girls in Iain's tennis class, has been talking about Chris for months. This evening while we were playing cards she called in with two friends, Lauren and Christa, fortunately with only ten minutes notice. Chris was tired, we'd been to see 'Catch me if you can' at the cinema and he had played a game of table tennis with Iain. Chris went white, then red when he was introduced but seemed to enjoy the visit even though most of their fast chatter was incomprehensible. It was Becca who kept the conversation going during their whirlwind half-an-hour visit. "Well, that's the first meeting over," said Becca. "That's always the most difficult." Iain teased him a bit about not saying much, and Chris coped, and then we went back to playing Hearts.

January 7th

Although he is moving away from a career plan of directing films, he watches all films critically.

We had been discussing yesterday's film. For lack of a better sounding board Chris has to use me. "Why does Spielberg go for the quick laugh, like the drunk being dragged into the street, in the pub scene between Leonardo and his Dad? It detracts from it." His ability to concentrate must be improving.

January 8th

We had a discussion today about school. Chris made it clear that he wants to delay starting school until August. "I want to go into a timetable that is as near normal as possible."

From my point of view the bulk of the teaching is in the autumn, which he has missed, and it would only be for the social contact that he would go now.

January 9th

Chris has bought an electric guitar with his Christmas money. Now we have to find a way to travel with it on the plane. We leave tomorrow.

January 21st

What dark days. Thank goodness for the guitar and the Strokes, and now Coldplay. Chris seems to have discovered a hidden talent and he plays for hours. This relieves me from trying to find things to pass the time, but it is horrible being stuck in this illness for so long.

January 31st

This has not been a good month. On the whole Chris felt quite good for most of the time that we were in the US. The warm weather must have helped along with a relaxed holiday atmosphere and company. We probably were not as careful as we should have been and failed to heed my own and other's advice. It is difficult to restrict activities when there have been so few occasions to enjoy. It didn't feel as if he was ill when, although he did very little, there was a life going on around us and each day was different. The mini holiday was basically one long car drive, but the variety was so invigorating for me as well as a distraction for Chris. I think that I was more disappointed than Chris that the ME recovery was not more. In all honesty I do not think there has been any. He has probably been more realistic about the month away, whereas I fell into the trap of thinking that it was all behind us because I was so much more relaxed. It was an illogical hope, wishing the illness to go away does not unfortunately mean that it will go away. Forcing the pace certainly doesn't work. I feel like crying all the time.

February 3rd

For the last fortnight Chris has had poor sleep and been cold and feeling bad. Apart from playing his guitar he has done no work and was unable to go to his English lesson.

"This is going on so long," I wailed to my mother on the phone. "This is such a bleak spell, especially after being in America. Chris is really paying for it and I am so scared that he might get worse again."

"Can you not go back to the Doctor, or the Consultant?" she asked.

"They can't help, they know so little, and all the Consultant recommended, you remember, was that Chris should go to a psychiatrist."

"Well, why don't you?" she queried.

I stopped my moaning rant abruptly. How could she understand when she had not seen us for over a year. I had invited her but she had declined, considerately, saying that I had enough on my plate. It is true, it is difficult trying to divide my time between guests and Chris. Perhaps she thought that Chris was depressed following our holiday. If she thought so, then how understandable it is for others to give him the same label. He may well feel low at the moment, I certainly do, but there is a wealth of difference between clinical depression and feeling down. I feel quite lost and alone as no one seems to be able grasp the complexities of this illness.

February 17th

Chris has had two guitar lessons. Today we had to cancel as, once again, it is freezing outside and he tells me his concentration is hopeless. He has had to stop the Maths with Andy because his brain fails to work however hard he tries. He has started to learn some Led Zeppelin songs.

February 27th

I rang the organisation who are running the film script competition to find out the results and they told me that they have extended the deadline.

March 1st

Chris still has not improved at all. February was a very sad month. His sleep is still poor although he does mostly sleep at night. He has not even played his guitar nor has he returned to have a lesson. Chris achieved an A for the essay that he wrote over Christmas for Mr Hart and he has had a couple of lessons since then. If I can not drive him he takes a taxi. He finds this very embarrassing but has weighed it up against the alternative, which is not to go at all.

> Do people have 'learned helplessness' with long term illness?
>
> Research form Chicago DePaul University suggests that people with a longer duration of illness, more than two years, were more likely to use coping strategies such as active coping; 'taking action to try and make the situation better', positive reframing; 'looking for something good in what is happening' and planning and acceptance; 'thinking hard about what steps to take'. This is in contrast to the opinion that patients develop 'learned helplessness'. Patients in the study were less likely to use behavioural disengagement or 'giving up the attempt to cope' which is seen in people ill for a shorter time.
> "It illustrates the indomitable power of the human spirit in coming to terms with a dreadful clinical and social situation."

March 3rd

At the Cross-Party group Alex heard about someone who examines Living Blood samples and treats with homeopathic medicine. We need to do something. I fear that we overdid it in USA but Alex thinks it was worth it to see Chris have some fun.

March 13th

Visit to Mr O'Hara, a homeopath. We were able to park within 150 yards of the clinic, which was a help as our consultation took over an hour. This is partly because it was so difficult to extract blood from Chris' thumb — Mr O'Hara said this was normal because ME patients were 'so bloodless'. Once the blood was on the slide Mr O'Hara looked at it for about ten minutes identifying parasites, red blood cells which he seemed to think were bunching together and the odd candida particles. I asked him why this could not be done by hospitals, and he replied that the live blood sample only lasts for about an hour. Chris has been given five different remedies to take including liquid oxygen and anti-parasitic pills. Some he takes for a month, others for two, when he will be reviewed. Chris was comfortable with him and commented that Mr O'Hara seemed to be really interested.

March 14th

The Film script competition results came in the post. Danny and Chris' script had been disallowed because of the violence implicit in the film when a bomb is heard to go off in the distance. This is particularly frustrating because there had been no such instructions regarding violence in the original rules. Chris was bitterly disappointed. For the last two years he has been analysing or discussing film and the various directing techniques. Winning the competition would have given him the chance to create a film and to judge his capabilities against those of his peers. This is something he has been unable to do at any level. If I am honest it is probably for the best because he would not be able to undertake the work necessary for the next stage. This is a reality that is hard to accept. As a consolation I bought him some Coldplay tabs.

March 15th

I have been looking for signs that Chris really is improving by comparing how he was two years ago. At last his room is untidy. There was a time when his room looked like a cell. Not a pen or book could be out of place, every video had to be in order and exactly in line. They say that ME people have a perfectionist personality but it is far more likely that as their brains struggle to keep some control, everything around them has to be organized. He can cope with light, and no longer do we sit in the gloom. On the whole his face is less spotty and his skin has some slight colour. His temperature control has normalised. He no longer dreads the hoover being switched on. Sleep, that ultimate bane of an ME's life is improving. He has spells of better quality sleep and he now sleeps mainly at night even if he still fails to fall asleep before 1 am. The most important aspect of it all is that his brain is recovering, especially his concentration, and this means that films and books are now so much more enjoyable. We take the ability to think rationally so much for granted that it is not a wonder that ME people think when this ability eludes them that they are going mad. This is why, I think, they need us around all the time. It is in order to help them make sense of their turbulent world.

March 18th

Chris is playing his guitar for hours at a time, despite having had no more lessons, and thus playing far fewer playstation games. He explained, "When I play the guitar I can feel my heart beat more slowly". The ME

Workshop in its monthly magazine reminds us that you have to include stress management as part of the healing programme. Music could be his.

April 4th

Jane has decided that I need a breather and we are going to the Lakes for two days. Chris probably needs a break from me too. Recently we met in the hall and each began to say exactly the same sentence. "We're just like an old married couple," Chris joked.

April 7th

There has not been much change with these pills. Chris had a sore throat for three days which, contrary to expectations, perked him up. During our consultation I told the homeopath that Chris never seemed to get colds or other minor illnesses. He explained that Chris' immune system is so low that you cannot really tell if he has another infection superimposed. So Chris sees this as a sign of recovery. Personally I think it is a reaction to staying with Danny for 24 hours. Neal is coming to Galloway for a couple of days while we are there for the Easter holidays.

April 22nd

Chris' 17th Birthday. I was really depressed this morning when Chris had almost no post and everyone seems to have forgotten him. Jane sent the usual cracking card and Jean never forgets. Gran came over for the day. Do ME patients become invisible? After their initial medical tests they rarely bother the doctor and once they have left school for a few months they disappear from the school register. They are not part of the working population and many do not or are not able to claim benefits. 'Sympathy fatigue' is understandable in long-term illness but I still am mystified that Chris only ever received one Get-Well card. I have to remember that I could have been as lacking in awareness in a similar situation. Jane's quirkiest card still hangs on the kitchen board. It says.

NEVER

NEVER

NEVER

GIVE

UP

Alongside it is one she sent while I was between jobs and before Chris became ill.

"How Nice It Is To Do Nothing And Then Relax Afterwards!" A bit ironic now!

April 23rd

My Birthday, and a really sunny day. I was standing outside holding a cup of coffee when Chris joined me. "Do you want some good news?" Of course I do. "My brain has been clear for a week." Perhaps after a month of O'Hara's pills appearing to do nothing, or even exacerbate Chris' symptoms, they are beginning to have some effect. Chris attributes this improvement to the liquid oxygen that he is taking. He says that it makes sense to help the red blood cells.

April 27th

At the Cross-Party Group this month there was a reception to launch Lynn Mitchell's book "Shattered', which relates the lives of twenty ME sufferers. Dr Vance Spence had come down from Perth. He is a vascular specialist whose organisation, ME Research UK, supported the publication. It gave me the opportunity to speak to him since I had never had a chance to thank him for his invaluable advice in the early days of trying to diagnose Chris' illness. "And how is your son coming along?" he asked. Dr Spence was having to sit down after the effort involved in travelling and speaking at the function. "He really is doing very well now," I was able to tell him. His gaunt, kindly face smiled up at me in pleasure and said, "He will get better because he has a mother."

May 6th

Chris has maintained his recent spell of better health for the last two weeks and our return visit to Mr O'Hara was today. He was to see if there was any difference in Chris' blood when he analysed it. I maintained a certain scepticism. Why, if he could see irregularities in the blood, could this not be done in a hospital environment? So, clutching the video of the blood test from the first appointment we arrived at the reception desk. The receptionist had no record of our appointment. Mr O'Hara was not even in town. The appointment is rearranged for Friday, three days from today.

May 9th

This time it was Chris who could not keep the appointment. Alex was not pleased but Chris is unable to do two trips in one week, especially as they were early in the morning. I rang to rearrange, again, only to find that Mr.O'Hara was returning to Australia. Fortunately, as Chris says, there is an improvement, but I feel rather let down.

Last year we had an equally exasperating situation when we needed to replace Chris' glasses - which had been sat on - and the frames needed replacing. The optician would only replace the frames if Chris had another eye test. It did not matter that Chris was housebound, and had not the energy to undergo a test, they were adamant.

May 12th

Work experience week. Danny had asked our neighbouring farmer if he could spend his work experience week on his farm. He and Chris spent the week in Galloway with Chris being in charge of meals. This arduous task meant remembering to put the stew or cottage pie in the oven at the right time. Chris had made an impact when he had first invited friends to stay by being the possessor of Wellington boots. The reaction to his decision to spend a week working on a farm had been equally incomprehensible to Danny's friends. At the end of the week he was vindicated. The farmer had paid him a good wage because he had worked so well. He became the envy of his group as he had been the only person who had earned any money.

May 19th

I have finally made an appointment with the surgery to have Chris' toe examined. I cannot believe how long it has been poisoned. It must be more than a year, and is probably aggravated because Chris is now wearing shoes. Our GP has given him some antibiotics. There is a risk that they will upset his gut but one we will have to take. He also has been given a chiropody appointment if he needs it.

May 26th

I notice how much better Chris seems while on the antibiotics and wonder whether a course would have made him better months ago. Then I remember all the courses that he was on before he became ill which made no lasting difference.

June 2nd

Our GP had once again, true to his promise of doing anything he could for Chris, written a letter endorsing the fact that we could not travel the thirty miles to attend an interview for the annual assessment of Chris' Disability Allowance. There was poor communication between their offices and the surgery. Despite his letter, I twice received letters informing me that we had failed to keep appointments made for us. This sort of bureaucratic time-wasting and harassment I certainly could have done without, but it gave us an inkling of the hurdles people face and their attendant anxiety when trying to access any form of financial assistance. We have an appointment for tomorrow.

June 3rd

This time Chris and I were more relaxed, mainly because Chris was, relatively, well on the mend. I defy anyone to say that he is fit for work, and indeed at present still could not attend more than partial schooling.

When the Doctor arrived I showed her into the conservatory. It was a sunny morning. Chris was dressed and wearing shoes - a far cry from the year before - but I was taken aback by the doctor's manner which was in sharp contrast to the gentle approach of the doctor who had done the assessment the previous year. She was business-like and took no time in telling us that she had questions to ask, no nonsense, no small talk. She certainly did not want any medical discussion, that was not her remit.

"So, Chris," she asked some time into the interview, "How do you spend your days, a typical day? You get up and wash?" she prompted. "Well, yes, and have breakfast." "You make your own and clear up?" "Well, no," I interjected, "I'm happy to do make his meals and tidy up so that he can use his energy for more useful things."

How could I explain what a zombie he was in the mornings and unless I placed breakfast in front of him he wouldn't eat for hours, and would feel awful? I could see her writing 'Mother attended throughout interview' and feel her disapproval at my not allowing a seventeen-year old to conduct an interview alone. But he could not. Sometimes his brain just would not filter all the information.

The Doctor continued, "And then what do you do?"

"Well, I watch T.V. or play the guitar."

"And after lunch?" she continued hopefully. Chris glanced at me briefly. I'd seen this look, years before, passing between a very sick teenager who was undergoing chemotherapy and her mother. That look could convey a whole message. Chris' look said to me, "Don't worry, Mum, she can't and doesn't understand, but I'm ok and don't worry."

"Well, I watch T.V. and play my guitar again. It's a bit boring really." She did not pick up on this telling observation, unable or unwilling to understand such a life, and ploughed on.

"And you see your friends and you'll be going to the cinema?" Chris nodded, while I wanted to add, "once a month perhaps."

"And you'll be driving soon and able to get around." This was a statement. I was stunned at her assumption that Chris would be given his own car but then I had been astounded at the closed questions that she had asked. Any self-respecting medical practitioner knows that all questions should be open-ended. It was with a sense of relief that she suddenly drew the interview to a close, and giving some unremarkable advice about his septic toe, she left.

June 16th
The effects of the antibiotics lasted three weeks. Chris' toe is poisoned again and I have made an appointment with a Chiropodist.

June 21st
We received the results of Chris' D.L.A. assessment. It has been disallowed. Out of a possible score of 10 he got 1. The point was marked against Mental Health. I am not telling Chris the reason. If he returns to school in August we will be able to claim Child Benefit again. On the AYME ability score he is now around 60%.

June 22nd
The Chiropodist has been very helpful, and has pared a lot of nail around Chris' toe. Chris now has to dress and bathe it every day.

June 24th
Chris and I both went into school to see the Director of Studies last week. We went armed with our proposal that Chris should join sixth year and study subjects that could be done in one year. I always promised Chris that he would not have to redo any year but would go back in with his friends. The Director readily agreed with all this. He said that he saw this year more as a testament to Chris' intelligence than with a view to entering University. We could negotiate that hurdle later. Chris would be unable to do a language or sciences because he has not the requisite grounding. We anticipated that by suggesting that he took Highers in History, English and Media Studies (the latter is only taken in sixth year and was an obvious choice). The Director added that he felt that Chris should add Intermediate 2 Maths. I explained that this was an area of Chris' brain still not functioning and we might jeopardise everything if he were to struggle with it. Chris explained to him. "I tried to do some maths last year but nothing made sense". All we had to do then, he advised, was to write a letter to the Headmaster with our decision.

How much exercise?

ME/CFS is a disabling disease which, despite numerous biological abnormalities remains highly controversial, wrote Twist and Maes. The bio-psycho-social model of management is adapted by many government organisations and medical professions to legitimise CBT and GET (graded exercise or adaptive exercise). Justified by this model GET is aimed at reversing deconditioning or muscle fatigue due to lack of use. Exertion using GET could well make a person worse and have a negative effect on patients. In Belgium CBT and GET have not been considered curative therapies since 2007.

Twist and Maes demonstrate that the success claimed for CBT/GET is unjust, and that it is unethical to treat patients with ME/CFS with ineffective, non-evidence based and potentially harmful 'rehabilitation therapies' such as CBT/GET. Exertion causes post-exercise malaise, extreme tiredness after exercise, because the effort involved may amplify the abnormalities in the patient's body that is causing their ME/CFS. The bio-psycho-social school of thought suggests that psycho-social factors are the driving force behind ME/CFS and are sustaining the illness and that the biological factors are far less important. The psycho-social-model had has its core elements that ME/CFS patients have a fear of movement, or exercise phobia and a personality disorder. Neither of these variants has been proved to be applicable in ME/CFS.

The reasons that GET is most likely to be harmful to ME/CFS patients are due to number of factors. This group of patients has a significantly reduced capacity of exercise, this group also 'recovers' from post-exertional malaise very slowly. In this group the ability of patients to recover takes over forty-eight hours (most people recover within twenty-four hours) and if they were asked to repeat the bout of exercise their capacity would be reduced by 25% - 30%.

The effects of exercise are not just limited to physical tasks, exercise seems to affect brain or neurocognitive performance. Also there is a decrease in the speed and impairment of working memory, which also requires a greater effort to be made. There is decreased blood supply with reduced oxygen exchange. This may be a possible explanation for the 'brain fog' reported by ME/CFS patients. Exercise also seems to reduce their Reaction Time.

Researchers show that structural damage to methods used by muscles to function and to the power house cells occurs in ME/CFS patients. These patients have impaired capacity to process muscle protein which cannot be explained by misuse. Exercise increases muscle pain and weakness and any kind of exercise can cause a patient to be incapacitated. The writers conclude that GET can physically harm patients with ME/CFS.

June 28th

The start of another summer holiday, our third. Chris is not dreading this quite so much. We are planning some driving sessions which we can start nearby because a friend has allowed us to practice manoeuvres on their private road. I am somewhat wary of Chris' ability to co-ordinate and assimilate all the information that is required to navigate safely.

July 1st

We are moving to a second floor flat just down the road from our flat in Edinburgh. In fact the bus stop for his school is immediately outside the door. We could never have contemplated moving from the ground floor before now. I hope it marks the end of the 'dark ages'. I know of one mother who has to carry her fourteen-year old up and down their stairs if ever they need to go out.

July 4th

So, in six weeks Chris will start school. We got a blazer and tie today at our second attempt. The shop is only twelve minutes walk away but last week he only managed to walk half-way. The vagaries of ME!

July 21st

We have got into the routine of going for a drive two or three times a week and combining it with a fifteen minute walk. The roads in Galloway are relatively quiet and in this way Chris can practise driving and get to explore the area that we live in.

July 23rd

This morning Chris asked if he could join his cousins in Cornwall.

"Why not ring now and ask them?" I replied while thinking, "Oh, help, please don't overdo it, not now, when you are so near restarting school."

Still, he has to begin somewhere balancing fun with caution. The train ticket is booked for 31st.

August 1st

Only three more weeks until school. I sometimes wonder whether Chris could have returned earlier. Certainly my enthusiasm for the idea at Christmas was misguided. Chris' cautious approach has proved much the wiser decision. Over the last months his condition has improved and stabilised, especially his sleep pattern. He has learned to 'live within his envelope of energy'. The test will be if this envelope is large enough to stand up to a school routine. To being, as Chris envisaged, as near as possible to normal.

August 24th
How strange that I can now talk of Chris' recovery in terms of months. Of how he has improved over the last months. In medicine we predict outcomes in terms of days or, at the most, weeks; so many days 'off sick'; so many days on antibiotics; so many weeks of chemotherapy; so many weeks in plaster. Rarely do we talk in terms of months, and never, in years. However after three years Chris is going back to school, albeit on a reduced timetable, but he will be attending every day.

August 25th
"How much is a pint of milk? I feel I ought to know these things."

August 26th
Start of term. The door buzzer rang while we were finishing breakfast. It was Danny. He called so that he could accompany Chris to school. A couple of other friends were waiting on the pavement outside the flat. I watched from the window as they walked in a small group down the street to the school and I could hardly believe what was happening. It felt a bit theatrical. I had been imagining it so often. Once again I had to bury my worries.

Chris had two days with his Media Studies group during the Festival. This helped to ease him in and enable him to reconnect with friends some of whom he had not seen for nearly three years. He had also gone to a "Chillies" concert in Glasgow the previous week where he met others of his year. He was elated when he returned from school. He had met boys who had had no idea where he had gone to, and been introduced to girls who said that they had heard about him. He was also greeted by members of staff who had taught him in third year.

Chris asked if I would mind going to Waterstones and buying him a copy of "Cal" by Bernard MacLaverty which they were to study for English. In with the book the assistant had slipped a bookmark. As I handed the bag to Chris I took out the bookmark and read:-
Never let your Schooling Interfere with your Education
Mark Twain

August 30th

Chris was invited, along with Alex and me, to the big family gathering and cricket match next weekend in Surrey. This is an annual event which we have missed for the past three years. He has decided not to come as he does not think the risk is worth it and he wants to keep a regular attendance at school. At dinner the night before the cricket match, David, his uncle, proposed a toast to Chris in his absence, congratulating him on his recovery. I wish he could have heard it.

September 15th

School routine is going well. Chris relishes both the lessons and the time in the common room during free periods. He seems to be valued for his talent for inventing common room games such as paper ball football. "I'm an expert in time-wasting games," he said, smiling. Having had a taste of company, the evenings and weekends are rather lonely. He knows he needs to rest at weekends so as to recover, but he also understands that it will take time to re-establish a place in his group.

September 22nd

A month of school now and Chris' health is steady and he is able to sleep. When nothing happened in his life I seemed to fill this diary because every small distraction from the boredom of waiting to get better was an event. Every day normal life, we are discovering, is full of distractions yet because it is common to every schoolchild it is not noteworthy. There is success in one essay, and disappointment in another. There is the anticipation of the result of an assessment or the organisation of a media project. All these make for a variety that we have not experienced for so long. There is a sense of excitement to each day.

October 5th

For several weeks just going to school was enough to make Chris happy. It was such a relief to have a routine and a positive proof of his progress. Gradually, however, he is realising that he has not slotted back into his year as he had hoped. Friends have regrouped, weekend habits have been established, as have music bands, teams for sports and free time activities. Through no conscious decision, but merely because he was never able to be included, Chris is forgotten.

October 9th

Chris rang one of his friends who he knew was meeting up in the town with others of his year. Immediately Chris was invited to join them. On this occasion he could and did, but he knows that simply completing his limited timetable is usually all that he can manage at present. He does feel a little sad when he realises how much he is still missing.

October 10th

October break. Alex and I are going to Spain with a large group of our friends, and Chris and Neal are going to Paris to stay with some cousins. I find it hard to remember now that there have been occasions in the last two years when I could see no point in holidays or in going away. I did not feel any resentment, just a lack of interest. Sometimes the brain is kind, and does not hanker after something that cannot happen. There were times when I would say to my mother on the phone, "my life is on hold until Chris is better," and sometimes I did say it in despair, but more for him than for myself - ask any other mother whose child has a long-term illness. The fact that other people are in worse situations does not make it any easier. It is just shocking that there *are* worse situations. We all want to be normal, and to think that a child would choose this sort of life as a manifestation of school phobia is inconceivable, but that is what has been said.

November 9th

Chris' toe is still not clearing. Fortunately, he is not taking games but he is planning to play cricket in the summer and there will be winter nets in the new year.

November 21st

The school routine and the way in which Chris' health has remained steady has reduced my constant state of anxiety as to whether we are pitching it right. I still have times when I fear 'what if ...', one of them being how will he cope with the increased pressure of work and the concentrated hours of prelim exams. We can keep the lid on his physical activities, but it is impossible to prevent the increased demand of studying for his three Highers.

December 1st

"Strokes" concert in Glasgow. Chris could not believe that they were coming to Scotland and that he was able to get two tickets. I drove him and Neal over and Helen came with me for company.

It may be fanciful but I shall always attribute much of Chris' recovery to this band and their music. Of all the music that Chris has listened to and learnt the Strokes have had the biggest influence on him. He modelled his wardrobe on them and has learnt all their songs. It is essentially such happy music. Chris has a shelf of mini-discs of music that he has recorded from the early months of his illness. To him they are a record of those years as vivid as any diary, yet he admits that he will probably never listen to them again, the memories would be too unwelcomingly powerful.

December 19th

The chiropodist has decided that part of Chris' toenail needs removing and afterwards he will need a week's rest. More rest! We know how we will all be spending this Christmas....

December 20th

I picked up a review of "The Strokes" concert that Chris has kept and which might explain their attraction. Andrew Perry wrote:-

Braehead Arena
"At a time when even Travis have been voicing political discontent, The Strokes rather gloriously brought nothing more than their music, their mundane songs of existential worry, uncertainty and ennui."

2004

"How pleasant it is at the end of the day
No follies to have to repent
But reflect on the past and be able to say
That my time has been properly spent."

Nursery Rhyme

Coping with disbelief is a burden that ME patients and their families learn to accept. They themselves have had to go through a journey of incredulity that they have an illness that is devastating and protracted and yet has no recognition or treatment. It does, however enable them to be understanding when this attitude is adopted by the lay person. This understanding is not always extended to the medical profession whom they resent because of their lack of interest and concern.

It is observed that once a patient accepts their own illness that sometimes they start to recover. This possibly refers to the energy that is expended in the stress of fighting a disease, especially an illness that is not accepted, which can then be directed instead to help with healing. Dr Speight reiterated the need for everyone around the child to believe what he or she said about his or her illness, again so as to reduce the stress that the child was under. For some members of the family, or for friends of the child who were seeing none of the day to day struggles, this would be a tall order. The innate trust in our health service - which, failing a diagnosis or treatment for the child, infers that there is a psychiatric condition - reinforces an outsider's belief in a psychiatric label. "It must be all in the mind." In other words, psychosomatic.

Children are well aware that they can be suspected of making things up. Chris at thirteen knew of this possibility when he accused the consultant of not believing him. When he grew older he, too, queried whether it could have been all in his mind. The physical symptoms were too varied and too unpredictable for him really to doubt however.

Unkind media coverage has fuelled the disbelief, with the terminology 'yuppie flu'. They contend that ME is an excuse for underachieving in a competitive world and write of a Headmaster who dubbed ME 'Mother's Excuse'. A kinder man, Dr James Fanu, wrote that there is a recurring pattern whereby doctors 'psychologise' illnesses they do not understand.

Could it be that the notion of a new disease is causing some of this disbelief? Or is it that ME is undergoing the same passage as other mysterious diseases such as Multiple Sclerosis which was dismissed as a hysterical condition? Why can there not be long-term childhood illness in this day and age? The picture of children confined to bed or wheelchair for months or years on end is not new. Clara, in *Heidi* by Johanna Spyri, recovered after years in a wheelchair; Colin in *The Secret Garden* by Frances Hodgson Burnett spent years in a darkened room — ME children will relate to that — and Marianne in *Marianne Dreams* by Catherine Storr was ill for months with an obscure disease. There is no saying that any one of them had ME, but the image of a child enduring a long illness is not new in literature and it is unlikely that these stories would have resonated with their readers if the premise was not essentially true.

Are there any tests or markers for ME?

Researchers in Miami have focussed on two potential markers for ME/CFS. The first is on natural killer cells, a type of white blood cell responsible for killing other cells and important for the body's defence against tumours and viral infections. Their function seems to be deficient in ME/CFS. The second is dipeptidyl peptise IV (CD26), an enzyme also involved in immune regulation and programmed cell death. The levels of this enzyme on white blood cells (lymphocytes) have shown to be increased.

The study shows that natural killer cells function significantly lower in 176 ME/CFS patients than in 230 controls. Also that the proportion of lymphocytes positive for CD26 was higher in ME/CFS than controls. These observations are consistent with the idea that an infection is involved in the initiation and/or the persistence of ME/CFS. The Miami researchers are now looking at how these levels change throughout the course of the illness.

February 10th

Chris is writing his second media studies film and it is exhausting him. Now the group are filming I had to contact his teacher and ask him to explain to Johnny, one of his film group, that Chris needs someone else to take over the organisation. The film includes quite a lot of their friends as actors and, unlike their last one which all took place in the flat, has several scenes set in and around the school. When there are so many strands to be linked up his brain seems to get overloaded.

February 13th

Chris is not working very much in the evenings. This dip in energy levels seems to stem from the Prelim exams. They were on consecutive days and drained him. He had been to see the guidance teacher and it was arranged that he would have extra time for each exam. What happens in reality is that, for example, both history papers are on the same day. The extra time is allotted at the beginning of every paper. He would start twenty minutes before the others, but then the break between the exams is shorter. There is less time to recover, and he ends up having a much longer day than the others. I feel that this term Chris has not recovered his energy levels. He had three days off soon after the exams with 'flu but I think it was a mild relapse.

The irony is that since he returned to school in August he has had fewer days' absence than he has had since primary school.

February 27th

More toe dramas, will it ever stop? Chris had to have the other side of his toenail removed. A great way to spend the February break! He then had to have another week off school to rest it and now has a month of dressings to do. The Chiropodist told Chris that the reaction he had last time was probably due to the phenol used as an anaesthetic when she removed the nail.

He has only been to a couple of 'nets' for cricket practice this term, and at the moment I am quite happy for him to miss them. He has not mentioned them either. As the cricket term looms it is becoming more and more imperative that his toe clears up. You cannot play cricket with an infected toe.

March 14th

This term has not been anything like as easy the last. Everything requires such an effort but I am hoping that a good break in the North Carolina sun with Iain and Becca at Easter will set him up for the exam term and cricket. Iain and Becca had twins early in January and we are anxious to see them. Chris is taking it sensibly at school and arriving late and leaving early as his timetable permits.

March 22nd

I never want to have a day like this again. I changed my hours this year enabling me to make sure that Chris has breakfast. I cannot see him bothering to cook sausages first thing in the morning! Then I leave for work once he has gone to school.

He is usually up and ready by eight but this morning he had not appeared. I knocked on the door and went in. He was still in bed. "I can't go to school," he said in a dull, flat voice. "My other toe has got infected." I didn't know what to say. I rang the absence line, gave him his breakfast and left.

On my way to work I thought I would ask the advice of my colleague at the Clinic. We could not go to our regular chiropodist because she was in Galloway. I needed help at once. Chris would be in the depths of despair. There is only a week until we go to the States and immediately after we return the cricket season starts at school.

"Is Karen in today?" I asked Lynda, our receptionist, as I arrived.

"No. What's up?" She seemed to sense I was upset. I explained about Chris' toe flaring up. It seemed so trite a matter but she left what she was doing and went over to the notice board. "She's not here until tomorrow, but why don't you try Felicity, here's her number."

How did she know I had to do something then and could not even wait until the lunch break? I had only once broken down at work and that had been two years before. They all knew that Chris was ill but I used work as an escape, only giving the odd update such as the great news that Chris was back at school. Felicity answered the telephone and said that she was sorry that she was working out of town but suggested that her colleague, Toni, might be able to help. Ten minutes later she rang back confirming that Toni would see us that afternoon and I was to ring at midday for directions and a time.

Toni said she was happy to stay on an extra half an hour and would see Chris at 5.30pm.

I rang the flat to tell Chris, but there was no answer. I rang the flat and his mobile before I left work but there was still no answer.

As I walked back through the centre of Edinburgh I felt as if my throat was constricted, a bit sick and weary. It was a resigned foreboding. Why didn't Chris answer the phone?

Was this it? Was this the point at which Chris would not be able to pick himself up again? Had he now lost hope of ever getting better? It seems rather dramatic now but as I walked through the park it did not seem so extraordinary to think that this could be it. Would this be the catalyst which tipped the delicate balance between hope and despair?

He was not in the flat.

I saw that his blazer had gone and a few minutes later a key turned in the lock.

"I decided I might as well go to school." he said.

Toni saw us in her clinic in Leith. She is pretty, attentive and painstaking. Even though she had been working all day including her lunch hour, we did not feel rushed. She treated his toe explaining it would quickly clear up. She explained that it had only reacted in this way in response to the uneven walking pattern he had developed while the other toe healed. One more treatment before we flew and he would be fine, she said, and she did not charge us. "Professionals should look after each other!" she said smiling.

As we drove away, Chris said. "Some people are just different, aren't they?"

> What has GENE analysis told us about ME?
>
> Genes are part of every cell in the body. A gene is a unit of heredity in a living organism.
> So far three systems in the bodies of ME patients are shown to be affected using gene analysis. Genes are either up-regulated or down-regulated in disease processes. In ME, the genes related to oxidation or the use of oxygen in the body, cell death (which is a normal process but which appears to occur too early in ME), and the immune system are either up- or down-regulated.

April 22nd

Chris' 18th Birthday. Alex and I took a group of Chris' friends out for a meal to thank those who had stuck by him throughout the three years, and to include his newly acquired friends. One such was Johnny, who, through their interest in Media Studies, shared a passion for film making.

"What happened to Chris?" asked Johnny, whose father is in the medical profession. "Did he get ill and then, just get stuck and not really want," ... he hesitated over the word as if it was not quite the right one, ... "to get better?"

May 1st

Chris got four runs and a catch in his first cricket match of the season. I'm staggered that they have put him in the team. He has not had any ill effects and certainly seems stronger after the break in the US.

May 7th

Chris can not manage the cricket training sessions as well as the matches and the coach is still letting him play. I expect he is well aware of the fact that he is hardly going to go in and score well after such a long gap and no practices. He just enjoys joining in at the moment.

The immune system in ME.

The immune system seems to play a key role in the pathogenesis (or cause or source of an illness) of ME/CFS. The immune system seems to be depressed while the inflammatory process is activated and this can adequately explain a number of abnormalities in ME/CFS. There is also a correlation between the severity of the inflammation and impairment with the severity of the patient's physical symptoms. Strenuous exercise is known to suppress some activities of the immune system and to aggravate some of the inflammatory processes even in healthy persons, and moreover muscles can be damaged.

Dr Klimas in Miami wrote that a large body of research supports the link between a disturbed immune system and CFS. A number of CFS symptoms are attributable to inflammation of various parts of the body such as muscles and joints. This has led some researchers to suggest that the immune system dysfunction causes the condition. Researchers have seen lower zinc levels, lowered omega-3 levels and raised omega-6, also defects in T-cells — all of which correlate with immune function. Oestrogen is an immune system regulator and levels of this hormone have been seen to be reduced. CFS rates are 2-4 times higher in women.

The best predictor of prolonged fatigue was the severity of the initial acute infection.

Long-term stress increases levels of substances which over time suppress the immune system. Natural killer cells are versatile white blood cells which can destroy infected cells. CFS patients often have reduced natural killer cell activity.

May 15th

The Higher History paper was today; all the others were taking the exam as a resit and were reasonably relaxed.

May 18th

Chris had a real struggle doing his Media Exams. His English and History exams were on consecutive days and there was only one day's interval before the Media exams today. He will be disappointed because Media is definitely his strongest subject and it has received the lion's share of his time.

May 27th

There is some subdued excitement and a fair amount of rivalry surrounding the forthcoming Battle of the Bands at school. Neal has encouraged Chris to play with his band and he has joined them on two or three practices at a studio in town. I think he had hoped to become fully part of the group but the band have been together for some time and realistically he is lucky to have a slot in their final number. Now there are the details to be decided upon such as what to wear and what to be called. All the others have stage names and Chris has to choose his. It seems it was an easy choice, he told me that he was just going to use Dougal's nickname for him.

"And what is that?" I asked

Chris gave me a grin. "Sickboy!"

June 8th

Last cricket match. It has been very disappointing for Chris that he has not shown any of his former flair for the game. Although it is to be expected, he has convinced himself that he never was all that good.

June 10th

Chris had been elated. He had worked so hard all week for the Showcase and was thrilled at winning the Media Prize. Yesterday evening when the repercussions hit and he realised that his energy is finite, he had to weigh up what he could manage. 'Yes' to the Sixth Form Ball. 'No' to the cricket. 'Yes' to his commitment to Media Studies. 'No' to going out that night. He looked crushed. It is wonderful when you look back to see how much Chris can do, but he is a long way from living a life compatible with that of his friends. It is very little consolation when so many activities are still beyond his capabilities.

June 12th

Jane and I are going to Sarajevo, Bosnia, for two weeks voluntary work. Somehow this is a statement. End of school, and end of me being in charge of Chris and his ME. Chris and his Dad are on their own. It seems unreasonable considering the progress he has made but I felt very sad for him last night. He said to me, "I just want to be well. Neal doesn't seem to understand that I can't do everything, like everyone else. I'm frightened I'll lose my friends over little things."

Would CBT have helped?

In the management protocol for ME/CFS using CBT and GET the Cognitive Behavioural model postulates that fear-based avoidance behaviour and physical deconditioning can explain many of the symptoms and impairments associated with the disease.

Dr Fred Freiberg of Stony Brook University in New York raised an important issue. Although CBT has a role in decreasing symptoms and increasing function there are considerable doubts whether avoidance behaviour and physical deconditioning are the causal factors in ME/CFS.

CBT facilitates the identification of unhelpful, anxiety provoking thoughts. It challenges negative automatic thoughts and their underlying dysfunctional assumptions. CBT combines a rehabilitative approach of a graded increase in activity with a psychological approach addressing thoughts and beliefs that impair recovery.

CBT is meant to eliminate the psychogenic 'maintaining' factors. Thus this theory proposes that by eliminating the maintaining factors of ME/CFS the patient can recover.

The proponents of CBT/GET derive their evidence from proven effectiveness in controlled trials.

Twisk and Maes examined the evidence to justify CBT/GET as a treatment for ME/CFS. They invalidated the bio-psycho-social model for ME/CFS and demonstrated that the success claim for CBT to treat ME/CFS is unjust. This model makes clear distinctions between predisposing factors (such as infections and trauma) and factors that maintain or sustain the disease (such as illness beliefs, stress, and inactivity).

In 2007 Bagnall in the York Review analysed all trials for CBT and /or GET and identified only 5 trials for ME/CFS using the Fukuda criteria. The others used the Oxford criteria which basically includes all people 'who present with disabling fatigue of uncertain cause' including those with diagnosed psychiatric disorders.

Solely based on fatigue scores the response to CBT was 40% in contrast to 28% in controls. Taking into account that fatigue is subjective and not measurable and is just one of the ME/CFS criteria, 'one can conclude that the effectiveness of CBT/GET in treating ME/CFS is non-existent'. 'Based on the evidence-based criteria and clinical experiences the claim that CBT/GET is the only effective treatment cannot be substantiated'.

July 2nd

Prize Giving and the last day of school. It is all rather unreal, partly because I have just come back from Bosnia, and partly because, in effect, Chris and his friends left school once the exams were over. It was strange to be watching what is a time honoured tradition without feeling in anyway part of it. I have had such a small amount of contact with the school. Chris and the other Prize Winners are able to choose their books and Chris has managed to leave his at the school. However, he will be back there over the next year. His Media Studies teacher has arranged for him and another girl to take Advanced Higher. Chris will also be working for the department when needed. A useful little job. It is difficult to see what else he could work at while he still needs flexibility regarding his health.

July 9th

Holidays officially start and Chris and two girls are heading with their tent to 'T in the Park'. It should be plain sailing now but these next months will not be easy, and the summer as ever is lonely if you are not fully fit and able to join in everything. To give him encouragement Danny has reminded him of their plan to travel and they are looking at starting in China next year. How strange that I have been writing all this time in a diary from The Republic of China 2000. The diary sits on the lower shelf of the telephone table in the Hall and I fill it in at random.

July 13th

Chris and I were walking towards Princes Street. He was heading to the music shop and I was heading for the bank. During our conversation Chris started to talk about what he might be doing this coming autumn. Then he said. "I never let myself think about the past and being ill, I'm frightened that if I do remember it, it will be …. sort of …. worse." Once it is over, or beginning to abate, the ME sufferer wants nothing more to do with the illness. They are ashamed at having a nebulous disease that has no recognition either of its impact or of its validity.

This remark reminded me of all those locked up memories on his shelf of mini-discs. I have been thinking that I should write out an account of it all. It would not only be for those who find the whole concept of ME impossible to understand, but also for him. It would be a record of his illness. Perhaps he will never read it.

July 15th

We have just been to an all-age twenty-fifth wedding party in Somerset, Chris' first social event. He was probably the youngest there but he seemed to suffer no qualms and always found someone to talk to. I nearly fell into the ME trap again of thinking that because Chris is doing normal things that life has returned to normal. The holidays loom and they present neither a chance to travel nor to stay with friends nor to work and Chris is adrift in no man's land. He feels abandoned and the loneliness is harder to bear after having had company every day for the past year.

August 1st

I went with Chris to buy him a full-sized keyboard on a hunch that his ability to play, lost in the early days of ME, might have returned. I justify the expense by calculating that a season's cricket with kit and travelling would probably have cost much the same. He's never mentioned joining his old cricket club again, and I have not brought it up.

August 7th

Chris is spending hours practising on the keyboard, and what with that, his guitar and the film world we seem to be limping through the days. To be fair I think I am more conscious of what he is missing than he is. He does talk of the difficulty of keeping up with friends, but he is always aware of how life was and chats enthusiastically about his plans for travel or his latest find on the music scene. Whenever I come in from work I invariably get "can you come and listen to my new" ... Led Zeppelin, Cold Play or Strokes, which he has just perfected on the piano or guitar.

August 8th

Exam results through today. Chris got two As and a B. The two As were a pleasant surprise; he is strong in History but he had not been so sure about English. The B for Media is a blow, but Chris recovered quickly after he had spoken to his housemaster. He remembered what a struggle it had been for Chris to do the exams that day and told him that his prelims count in an appeal. He is going to ask for one.

September 3rd

Sussex. A village green. One of those wonderful days. Sitting in the sun in the Pavilion or walking around the boundary, surrounded by friends and family. Alex, Dougal, Chris and Iain all playing cricket at the annual end-of-season gathering. Chris was so happy and everyone made such a fuss of him. He did not have much of an innings but to be part of the team is an achievement in itself. The last time he had been here had been five years ago when he was thirteen. He was strictly too young to take part then, but the opposition had been short of a cricketer and he had been allowed to play.

September 7th

At School special arrangements have been made for Chris to do Advanced Higher Media. This keeps a link with the department and a focus for the year. Chris will also have the chance to earn a bit helping the Department. Chris' housemaster, who has organised this, must have an extraordinary understanding of the void that Chris is facing by offering to take him through another Higher. It is an area he can develop if he finds he can not get into any University.

September 17th

Now that child benefit has stopped Chris has no money that he can call his own, I have devised a scheme of things he still is not happy to do and putting a value on them. He can 'earn' by doing such things as ringing to book driving lessons, going to have his hair cut [it's the chat], type out a letter for me, or hoover. This is until he starts earning by working in the Media department.

What is POTS?

POTS is Postural Orthostatic Tachycardia Syndrome, or fainting or feeling faint when standing. ME patients suffer from this. They are unaware that they feel so ill just from standing up. One of the causes seems to be the pooling of blood in the lower limbs. Normally we have systems in place which prevent our blood vessels dilating and the blood pooling when we stand up, but this does not happen in ME patients, and as a result they feel faint and their heart rate goes up. Their lower limbs and feet become swollen and blue. This is why some patients use wheel chairs. If they are more sick then they have to lie down. Some ME patients drink copious amounts of water in an effort to increase the volume of their blood. In a recent study of a 20yr old girl with severe ME who undertook treatment with Prof. J. Newton in Newcastle, 25mg of atenolol, increased fluid intake and daily tilt table training saw improvement in a year to her being able to do almost daily outings.

October 1st

Chris was awarded an 'A' on appeal for his Media Higher, which made him very happy and his brothers very annoyed. 'Now Chris can boast that he's the only one with straight As.' The school are helping Chris with university applications and especially with his personal statement which will tell them more about him than his results.

October 4th

The effect of a diagnosis of ME was reiterated this week when I spoke to the parent of a dancer who I had been treating for painful knees. Her mother told me that her daughter had been diagnosed with depression, but, with another slant put on her symptoms, they fitted those for ME. I suggested the possibility that, as her symptoms were exacerbated each year by exercise, had the doctor considered any other diagnosis? To my surprise she answered almost aggressively "Are you talking about ME?" And before I could say anything she was on the verge of tears and outraged as she continued "How can you think it could be ME, I know about ME and isn't it better to have depression, which Doctors can *do* something about?" I was shaken by her vehemence. Hers was a reaction of utter rejection, as if I had said cancer. Yet how could I have forgotten my own equally dismissive reaction to Alex's suggestion years ago that Chris might have it? I had managed to bury the thought until the facts were too plainly in front of me. The diagnosis fills you with such dread that you can forgive all the medical practitioners who delay a diagnosis until there is obviously no other.

Dougal told me that the parents of one of his pupils had discussed the possibility of her having ME. "If you ask a person all that list of questions about their symptoms, will it not suggest symptoms to them?" He challenged me. My answer was to tell him that this is one of the perennial questions. It seems to raise its head when the interrogator is sceptical of the subject. The answers to questions on other medical problems are not doubted in the same way.

October 7th

Chris is spending hours playing the piano. He was about to take Grade I when he last played, and here he is playing a piece that would stretch someone of Grade 7. He does work out the notes, but after that he seems to use a combination of memory and intuition especially when it comes to timing. It is not as though he is doing it by ear and that he has heard the music before, which I could understand. It is as if he has bypassed the analytical part of music reading and gone straight to an area of his brain that does it for him. He did the same with the guitar tabs. He still has to do hours of hard application but the results are exciting.

October 15th

Alice, whose son had ME on a parallel course with Chris, went to a Conference of the Royal College of Paediatricians and Health Care.

CFS was on the agenda and Dr Nigel Speight invited to speak. He has supported many families through the horrors of child protection. He pointed out how poor the research is in ME, especially with children. He emphasised that children are ill with so many sensory symptoms that fatigue is the least of their complaints.

Alice felt reasonably positive about most of the speakers but was discouraged to find that the discussion focussed on child protection, mother's harmful influence, home tuition causing entrenching of the illness, MSBP, and using ME to commit benefit fraud.

Alice pointed out to the conference that if mothers were overprotective then it was to protect them and their children from suspicion, disbelief, forced exercise, forced schooling and child protection orders. The idea of benefit fraud was nonsense since ME patients find it so hard to access *any* benefits. She left dispirited by the huge change in attitude still required, especially as she could envisage no other childhood condition where child protection would be the main topic of open debate.

October 16th

That was an unnerving experience! Just when I thought that the ME was fading into the background. Chris has been doing a lot of editing, working on his media studies, and learning new music pieces recently. Alex and I are going to Bath for a few days. About 8.30 in the evening as I was finishing my packing. I went through to say something to Chris. He looked strained. He was lying on his bed, the TV was not on, and he asked if I would just stay for a while. I suppose it was what they call a sensory storm. He felt totally detached from reality and he was extremely scared. It lasted about four hours and we talked a bit and I just sat beside him and waited. It was as if all the worst symptoms, the brain symptoms, had struck all at once. It finally settled down and Chris said it was all right for me to go.

October 21st

There was an advertisement on the door of the Clinic, when I went into work today, for a part-time receptionist. "Chris could do that." I found myself thinking, "but would he want to work with me, and would they want him?" I asked the senior physiotherapist if she would mind if Chris applied. They had never had a male receptionist before but she said she was happy to interview him. Although it is not very cool to work in the same place as your mother, our shifts would rarely overlap. When

I told him about it Chris said that "if it's the chance of a job I'll give it a go." He has no idea what it entails because he has never been to the Clinic. I am amazed at how calmly he took the idea.

November 6th

A week until Chris' driving test and we have been going out a bit more often in the car to enable him to have some extra practice. I am a bit disturbed. Driving along one of the major roads leading out of the city, where there was very little traffic, we came up behind a bus. It stopped to allow passengers to alight. Chris pulled out slightly. I could see one car coming towards us, about a hundred or more yards away.

"Can I overtake?" he asked.

"Up to you." I replied.

"Well! Tell me whether I can or not," he snapped, "you know I can't tell distances."

November 13th

Chris failed his driving test. He did, however, get the job.

November 15th

Life is pretty good now and very busy with school work to fit in as well. Weekends are still quiet but on Wednesday evenings all his friends meet up in town and he joins them. He makes sure that he does not organise a shift at work for the Thursday morning .... especially as he will often go back and spend the night on someone's floor.

November 16th

Chris is becoming increasingly perturbed by Danny's reluctance to commit on their trip to China, Australia and New Zealand. I really do not think he will pull out but Chris has arranged with the school to be away for the spring term and time is getting short. I don't know why Danny is being elusive about it and I don't think, this time, that his girlfriend is the problem.

November 18th

Danny has called up Chris and they met to discuss China. There was, or is, a problem. Danny's great friend Hayworth wants to join them. He was planning to head to Australia too, but his travelling companion has fallen through. Hayworth is a rugby player and one of the stronger characters in their year. Chris holds him rather in awe and I remember him because of Danny's 16th party. The party was held at his house and he had urged Chris to go to for a short while. When he returned, excited at meeting so many people, he had mentioned that Hayworth had been particularly friendly, and had gone out of his way to make him feel part of the group. Now they need to decide whether to include him, although I expect that it is an easy decision.

November 28th

I had one of those bad nights when you are suddenly wide awake at 2 am and your brain starts churning. Chris is doing so much and trying to finish school projects. It is crazy. Yesterday he told me, "When you shut your eyes it's black. I use that to get to sleep when my brain is spinning. This time it was white. I wrote it down. This morning on my text it said 'I can see white.'" I suggested that he drop the driving lessons for a while and cancel his re-sit test. He must be overloading his brain, which seems to need time to recover its full function.

November 30th

Chris had an easy day at work, just filing. In the evening his brain felt clearer than it had for ages and he got the plan of an essay, which had been plaguing him for days, done in twenty minutes.

"I think the physical side dictates the mental. There is a mental side to it but only when I'm tired. Is that ME or is that normal?"

"Normal, I think, but more pronounced in ME," I replied.

"Now when I have a bad spell I seem to come out of it better."

December 1st

Chris, Danny and Hayworth are in constant contact and the trip is booked for Jan 14th starting in China. All those months of tedium are forgotten.

December 21st

For the last two Christmas breaks Dougal and Katie have worked for the homeless serving meals and giving out clothes at CRISIS. Chris has asked to do a day with them. This year it has been organised in the Dome. After that we are all spending Christmas together.

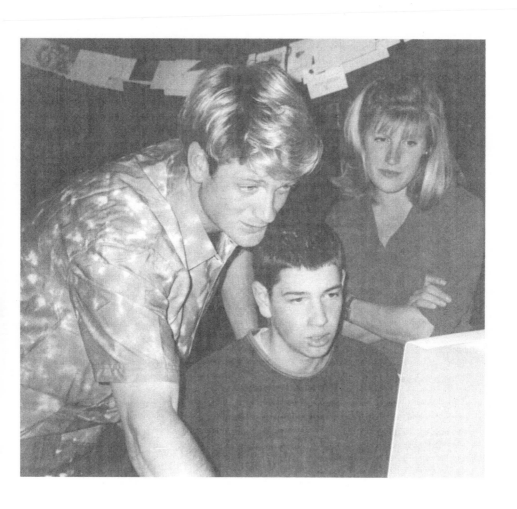

2005

So why do I think Chris recovered? The natural course of ME, with no interventions, is known to be around four and a half years. Recent research has indicated that an unsympathetic approach from GPs in the early stages tends to mitigate against an early recovery. This is a harsh statement because, as can be understood from the conflicting evidence with which doctors are presented, they have guidelines encouraging them to treat the condition with a psychiatric management programme. In most cases their own knowledge from medical books and journals is scarce.

ME can have a sudden onset, with what resembles an acute infection which fails to resolve, or it can have a gradual onset. Chris seemed to have a combination and the duration of his gradual onset episode started in effect from 1997 and he was only fully recovered by 2007. Even now he could not pursue a sporting career and has only a limited capacity for physical exercise.

Chris was anxious to help himself and diet seemed a low risk approach. From the outset I was convinced that Chris was suffering from an illness with an organic basis and I never at any time saw evidence of depression. Despite the criticism that ME has 'too many symptoms', it was this aspect that was the key factor that confirmed in my mind that ME was what we were dealing with. I think that Chris' ME just ran its course.

ME patients try a myriad of treatments in an effort to get better. Some have used the Mickel Reverse therapy which is a talking-based therapy that helps to correct the over activity of the hypothalamus gland, or the Lightning Process which is a combination of life coaching, self-hypnotherapy, neuro-linguistic programming. and osteopathy. Others have tried postural hypotension training (POTS), and probably many others, but no one would be able to say for certain that these approaches cured them, and none of them have consistently good outcomes.

People will do anything in order to regain their health. They will endure chemotherapy, amputations, harsh rehabilitation regimes and restrictive diets, if they believe they will help. Iain told me of one man in North Carolina with ME who recovered by eating only melon for a month. Yet not recovering from ME is not due to not trying, or not finding the right treatment. No treatment cures ME. It is not fair to blame, be irritated with, or dismiss as uncooperative or not trying, any unfortunate person who fails to recover. These people are the most in need of empathy, care, benefits and research for a cure.

January 13th
The Hayworth family invited us to a send-off meal for Danny, Hayworth and Chris before setting off for their three month trip to China, Bali, Australia and New Zealand. They were given matching t-shirts and posed for the obligatory photos.

YOU CAN PUT THE BOY OUT OF SCOTLAND,
BUT YOU CAN'T PUT SCOTLAND OUT OF THE BOY.

January 14th
One of the Universities, Chris' first choice, contacted him two days before he left to ask for an example of his work. There was a rapid exchange of emails between him and Dougal because the formats are incompatible. Dougal said that the work was a little ragged around the edges and that he and Katie had tidied it up so that it was well presented. He forwarded it on today.

February 2nd
Results are coming in from some of the Universities that Chris has applied to. One was a refusal because Chris has no music qualification on paper. One is no longer running the course. Three have offered him places. The other, the one that he would most like to go to, has called him for an interview.

I rang and said that he was in Australia.

February 20th
Chris was given another interview date. I rang and said that he was in New Zealand.

March 3rd

A post card has arrived from the University to say that because Chris could not attend the interviews they were unable to offer him a place.

March 15th

Chris and Danny have e-mailed to say that they have decided that they aren't going to University. I think they plan to travel for ever and start working. Although Chris' decision does not affect us, it will be very upsetting for Chris' housemaster who has put in so much time and effort into helping Chris with his advanced higher. I asked him to email his housemaster himself.

An excerpt from Chris' e-mail.

"I was concerned that the results of my Highers would not gain me a place at University. I never thought that my health would have held up as well as it has. There has been no sign of ME. When I returned to school I made a decision that were I ever to have a relapse of ME I would have packed as much into my life as I could until that day. Out here I finally feel like I've been doing it ....without wanting to sound overly corny I could never have imagined how happy I have been over the past eight weeks."

Chris' Housemaster gave me a copy of his reply.

"Thanks very much for your letter which explains your position fully. I accept its reasoning and clarity outright and please don't worry about making it. It's your life and only you can live it. It is always a difficult situation where three dangerous elements are put together in the world ... and I don't mean you, Danny and Andrew; rather youth, opportunity and the freedom to decide. I admire you for making the call and having the insight to determine what you do, rather than let it be determined for you, as too many of the kids here continue to do and I did myself at your age but in different circumstances.

You are doing absolutely the right thing if that is how you feel and you are happy; an elusive state at the best of times. I wish I had had the courage to make such a decision at your age. Good Luck.'

March 17th

I met up with Davina's mother today. As usual we went over the same old ground, always wondering if we could have done something that could have enabled our children to recover quicker, or to have prevented the deterioration in the first place. She tries not to feel angry that the prescribed exercise in the gym made Davina so much worse, because she knows that it is unhelpful when trying to focus on the future. Her anxiety is that, as mentioned by one of the doctors that they have seen, the cells' mitochondria (the power house of the cell), could be permanently damaged. We also go over all the possible routes to recovery that we hear about, or read about, but they all entail risks that we are not prepared to take. So we both play the waiting game. There is no denying the fact that Chris is making progress, where Davina is not, and that the only difference is that she was encouraged to undertake a regime of exercise.

March 21st

I attended the Cross-Party Group where Chris Clark, the Chairman of AFME (Action for ME), was speaking. Research into CFS alone is objected to by the ME self-help groups because they believe that ME is a distinct illness in its own right and that it should not be absorbed into the umbrella term of CFS. Often people who consider that they have ME then find out that they are suffering from a recognised disease such as Lyme Disease, or Airline fuel fume toxicity, or Coxsackie's virus, and so on. On the other hand those with Gulf War Syndrome, Organophosphate poisoning or Multiple Chemical sensitivities will know that they are not suffering from ME, but neither do they feel that they should be under the umbrella of CFS. It is because so many conditions have been clumped under CFS that these groups are antagonistic towards psychiatrists, Adding to the antipathy is the fact that trials for treatment for CFS are on patients who usually have a mental condition. For patients with mental conditions the treatment regime seems to be successful but then the results of trials with that group are thought to be beneficial for everyone that has been labelled CFS. There is a need for all these separate groups to be researched individually.

Chris Clark had a frosty reception. He did not help himself by talking about 'harmful advice given out by some self-help groups which actually encouraged people to rest in the toxic phase, whatever that is.' As he was quoting from guidelines set out by ME Association, advice which everyone in the room would agree with, it was no wonder that he had an unsympathetic audience.

April 5th

We had a long phone call from Chris early this morning, very long, and we could tell that something was bothering him. Hayworth had returned to Sydney the week before. Then Danny's grandmother had died, and he had flown home around the same time. Chris had decided to try travelling on his own, and was staying with friends of Alex's in North Island, but we could sense he was lonely and travel weary.

"Why don't you just come home?" we suggested.

Chris will be home in a week.

April 13th

While Chris was making tracks to return to the UK, Iain was organising his brother's future at University. Apparently the Department had rung and offered Chris another interview and Iain had accepted on his behalf and arranged a date. Knowing when Chris was due to land in London he arranged the interview for the following day.

What he did not appreciate, and nor did we until he arrived, was that Chris' journey took 55 hours due to a long stop-over in JKF. The joy of student flights. On his flight from Los Angeles to JFK he had had nothing to eat because he had no dollars. In JFK he had been sitting, hopefully having found some food, for about four hours when a fellow traveller sitting beside him turned to him and said, "I hate this waiting around".

"How long have you got?" asked Chris.

"About eight hours, how about you?"

"About twenty-two!"

Dougal met him at the airport and told us later that Chris stank. His hair was shaggy and he had grown a beard. Dougal said that he did not know what they would think at the interview, but Chris said he needed sleep more than a haircut.

He is catching an early train tomorrow morning and sounds remarkably alert.

"I feel, Mum, that now I've got an interview, I've got a good chance. I'm reasonably confidant that I can get in if I can just talk to someone."

April 20th

Chris did talk his way to a place. At one point they asked him whether he had more examples of his work and he told them he was lucky to be able to do what he did. They seemed to accept that. The interview was followed up by a phone call and Chris was asked if he thinks he will manage the course. He was unlikely to say no. Now we know that he is settled for September.

May 7th

ME Awareness Day. Alex was interviewed after the reception at the Parliament. The report was captioned 'Give Us Strength.' He was asked. "What are the people with ME doing, themselves, to raise awareness of their problems? Why were they not congregating and demonstrating if they felt that there was an injustice.?"

Alex: "Well, that is the problem … they don't have the energy to do either."

June 16th

I have just returned from two weeks work with Jane in Sarajevo. Today Chris and I had dentist appointments. It is a silly landmark but he hasn't been for nearly five years. The sugar-free diet must have had a dual benefit because along with helping his recovery he does not need any fillings.

June 17th

Davina and her family are holidaying near by and we asked them all over for a BBQ. Davina knows that we understand if she needs to disappear to rest on the sofa at any time. I wonder if we were like them when Chris was so ill. The natural spark that ignites when people meet socially was there but very subdued. I wonder too, if Iain and Dougal had been younger and closer in age to Chris, whether they would have been affected in the same way as Davina's two sisters. Perhaps feeling guilty that they are well, perhaps not wanting to capture the limelight and leave Davina neglected, they were relatively quiet. "Did you notice," Chris remarked afterwards "that all Davina's conversation was about other people, what they had done or were doing, and also what an effort she made." Alex found great empathy with her father, whom he had not met before. "He's doing what I did, he just works all the time. You just don't know what to do."

August 19th

There has been a call for physiotherapists to help our advisors on the National Institute for Health and Clinical Excellence (NICE) guidelines. I had offered to help but it is impossible to download the information as the reading is enormous and the average home computer cannot manage. The Canadians have brought out their own guidelines which are excellent but at a hundred and nine pages still too long for a GP. The Australian's are only seventeen pages and also good. There are so many circulating around already and the fact that they differ very little from each other shows the paucity of real information. None of them give any space to recent physical research results.

August 23rd
A recent headline in *The Times*:
Yuppie Flu
It may not be all in the mind - it might be in the genes.
Chris is rather partial to this nomenclature 'yuppie' he tells me.
The article is referring to the exciting research into genes. Both Dr Gow in Glasgow and Dr Kerr in London have identified genes that are overactive in the areas of the immune system, oxidative stress and high levels of apoptosis or cell death. The hope is that one day, not only will this lead to possible treatments but more immediately, to bio-markers or tests for the illness.

September 22nd
The problem of vaccinations, again. Chris needs to have a BCG and Meningitis jab before going to University. When I booked them at the surgery the nurse said that she would ask the Doctor to contact me since I was concerned. BCG has been known to trigger ME. The Doctor rang back as soon as he had finished his surgery. Apparently the BCG is no longer compulsory, and the meningitis is a dead vaccine therefore unlikely to cause a reaction.

September 24th
Chris has not been feeling well since his jab two days ago and was understandably anxious. "I hope it wasn't stupid having the injection, that I didn't do it because I was just doing what they told us to do. It was sensible wasn't it? At least I can still write. I've done two pages. I can type quickly enough to keep up with my ideas and with the words the way I want them to be."

September 28th
Chris soon recovered from the jab. He has been very busy getting ready for University where he will be staying in a student house. Some of his belongings are in London but all the rest had to fit into a rucksack, except for his guitar and his computer.
Alex and I took him to the airport and stood back as he checked in.

I recognised the person who was checking him in. "That's James, do you remember, from Croy farm, they used to travel to school together every day." James kept Chris guessing as he checked him in. It had, after all, been five years since they had seen each other and James had the advantage of having Chris' name on the ticket. The chance meeting gave us an easy topic of conversation before we had to wish him a cheerful goodbye.

September 30th
Chris rang today to say that he'd settled in to his Uni-house but had had to borrow covers and a pillow because we hadn't thought about him needing any bedding.

October 18th
Alex and I are visiting Iain, Becca and Sam and Lucy in the States and we have had a rather forlorn phone call from Chris. He has a cold, the initial excitement has worn off, the forty minute walk to college is a bit of a killer and nearly all the other uni-lets are much nearer the campus. Becca was so concerned. "I hope that I haven't raised his expectations too much." But we decided that it was probably too many late nights and trying too hard to keep in budget and not eating properly. Also he had been along to the first nets. I think he realised that cricket will never now be part of his life; unfortunately there is no substitute for the years of experience that he has lost.

November 1st
Chris on the phone and everything is rosy. Someone in his study group suggested that they all meet up for a drink and this has opened the gates for all of them to expand their contacts. Chris seems to have found a fellow guitarist.

November 5th
We have had an unexpected chance to visit Chris at University. Alex and I had to go down to a funeral about ten miles from the town. He is full of enthusiasm and playing a bit of football, "I think I pack more into my week than anyone else!"

December 12th
Christmas can be very dull once the family has dispersed. Our present to Chris is an air ticket so that he can spend a fortnight with Iain and his

family in the States. By leaving before the rush he has found a reasonably priced flight. We should catch a glimpse of him just before the next term starts.

December 30th

Chris told me that his close friends now know about his ME. One of his two particular friends got diagnosed with diabetes two weeks after arriving at the University. The third friend now feels that he is the odd man out! This is a marked change from even a few months ago when he didn't want any more do to with ME let alone admit that he had had it. This was illustrated by an incident that happened two days before Chris started at University. He rang and asked if he could meet me for a coffee. Why? I wondered. We saw each other all the time.

"Can we not just talk on the phone?" I asked him.

"Well, it's not easy." He replied. So I waited a few moments. "It's about this book you're writing. I know you're writing it and I don't want you to." It was true. I had started it when he had left for China.

I waited again.

"There was this programme where two parents were psychiatrists and they had written a book about their daughter and her condition. They were all being interviewed and they were analysing her ..." He trailed off.

"I promise that you will never be involved." I told him. I did not promise that I would not go on writing it because the ME story needs to be told, but it should be possible to protect him, especially now that he has left school and leads his own life.

Diagnoses and Misdiagnoses

"Dost thou love life? Then do not squander time
For that is the stuff life is made of."

Benjamin Franklin

There are no records as to how many people in Britain have ME but there are indications of the numbers from a variety of sources. The CMO report said that the incidence of CFS/ME is 0.2-0.4%, around one in every five hundred of the population. This is at least 125,000 CFS/ME patients in UK. In comparison, there are 100,000 type 1 (insulin-dependent) diabetics and 100,000 multiple sclerosis sufferers.

In a snapshot of the incidence of ME in Scotland two areas were surveyed in 1998. Two hundred and thirty-six cases were found in Fife and sixty-five in Wester Ross. The similarities in the two surveys were striking. In both surveys the incidence peaked between the ages of thirty and sixty with ten per cent being below the age of twenty. The average duration of the illness was four to six years but fifteen per cent had symptoms ten to twenty years later. Fifty per cent of the patients rated themselves sixty to seventy per cent disabled. In children the onset for boys was under twelve and it was over twelve for girls. In Fife fourteen percent had another family member with the illness. In Wester Ross the figure was eleven per cent.

When Jane Colby and Dr Elizabeth Dowsett compiled a survey in 1997 of one thousand and ninety-eight schools involving 333,024 pupils they found that fifty-one per cent of long-term medically confirmed sick had ME. The fourteen- to sixteen-year old age group was hardest hit, but the survey showed that children as young as five had the condition.

When in 1997 Dr Bell followed up an outbreak of over two hundred cases that had occurred in his practice in New York in 1984 he found that of the twenty-four girls and eleven boys who had fallen ill with ME only thirteen had had a full recovery. Of the rest, fifteen were well but had not fully recovered, four were chronically ill and three were more ill than during the early years of their illness.

ME is complicated in every aspect of its presentation. It has so many symptoms that some doctors argue that the patient must be fabricating them. ME does not fit into easy parameters where the main features can be gathered together to provide a recognisable entity. In an effort to simplify and encapsulate what ME is for research or clinical purposes essential criteria have been selected by different organisations.

To do research, scientists have to be able to accurately identify on which patients they are conducting the research, and for this there has to be a specific label or diagnosis. There are at least four criteria that have been produced to describe the patients suffering from CFS/ME.

In 1991 and 1994, respectively, the Oxford and the Fukuda Criteria described CFS/ME with fatigue as the principle symptom. The fatigue had to have had a specific onset, have been present for at least six months, and it had to be disabling to physical and mental functioning fifty per cent of the time. Other symptoms could be associated with it such as muscle pain, joint pain, headache and sleep disturbance.

The US Centre for Disease Control (CDC) updated their Criteria in 1994 and added that four of the following should accompany the fatigue. Post-exertional fatigue, impaired memory or concentration, unrefreshing sleep, muscle pain, multijoint pain, tender neck or axilla nodes, sore throat or headache.

Finally in 2003 the Canadian Criteria was produced. This was much more satisfactory as far as ME patients were concerned, since many of them do not rate fatigue as their most disabling symptom. The Canadian Criteria described post-exertional malaise and fatigue of six months duration, sleep disorder, pain and neurological or cognitive manifestations. They added that at least one symptom from two of the following systems had to be present. These were symptoms from the autonomic, neuroendocrine or immune systems. Autonomic symptoms are those such as orthostatic intolerance (feeling faint), extreme pallor, intestine disturbance (irritable bowel), bladder dysfunction or palpitations. Neuroendocrine symptoms are those such as loss of temperature control (feeling hot when in a cold environment or vice versa), anorexia or abnormal appetite, and loss of adaptability which worsens with stress. Immune symptoms include tender lymph nodes, sore throats and flu-like symptoms, general malaise, development of allergies such as to alcohol, and hypersensitivity to chemicals or medications.

Although this new and acceptable criteria is helpful to discerning doctors, it has not been the criteria used for research purposes. The broader scope of the former criteria has been used which means that conditions other than ME are included. In fact all unexplained fatigue states are included and this inevitably includes mental health conditions.

So far, in Britain, there are no separate criteria for children. In the US Jason and Bell adapted the Canadian criteria with special emphasis for children. They advocate that a diagnosis be made after three months. Although the diagnosis is not particularly helpful from the point of view of treatment options, because as yet there are none, they say that it relieves the child of other labels such as school phobia, which may be more detrimental to the child and its family. They explain that the physical fatigue may be manifested as behavioural irritability and the mental fatigue as the child being easily distracted. They suggest that a measure of severity be placed against symptoms which fluctuate regularly so as to monitor progress, and that more than one close adult helps with the symptom list so as to gather a more rounded picture of the child.

The classification of an illness is an important issue because since 1969 ME has been classified as a physical neurological disorder. At one point in its history CFS/ME found itself classified under mental health disorders as well. The World Health Organisation ruled that CFS/ME could not be classified twice and endorsed the original physical label. It was due to this polarisation of medical opinion that the Chief Medical Officer (CMO) decided to commission a report into CFS/ME the results of which were published in 2002. Dr Speight, who believes in the physical aetiology of ME, was on the advisory group for children and young people. He could see from the deliberations that, if ME was placed under mental health, his own job would have been on the line as he had already diagnosed some two hundred children with ME.

The future for many ill people hung on the results of the CMO's report. Even before it started, however, the ME support groups voiced their concerns regarding the members of the commission that had been appointed. There were three committees which were made up of a working group, an advisory group of people whose interests were children and young people, and a reference group. The working group was made up of doctors, patient support group workers, and carers. The doctors were predominantly psychiatrists with well known views as to their belief that CFS/ME was a mental condition following some infection of unknown cause. It was this that concerned ME support groups.

The second area of concern was that the working party was directed only to look into best practice treatment and management and not into the cause, prevalence, or possible lines of investigation into CFS/ME. In fact the report when it came out stated that only basic and limited tests were appropriate, and specifically that there was no need to perform immunological and neuro-imaging investigations.

Towards the end of the working party's deliberations it became apparent that the outcome was not emerging in a form that pleased the psychiatrists and the majority of them walked out. Although there were calls for the report to be published in their absence, there needed to be clarification and endorsement of the classification of ME under neurological disorders and that it was not moved to a classification of psychiatric disorders.

The press hailed the publication with enthusiasm for the medical establishment's acceptance of ME as a 'real' disease.

The CMO report stated that CFS/ME is relatively common but lacked specific markers. It said that the cause is unclear but that the impact of even a mild form can be extensive. It stated that current evidence does not distinguish CFS from ME, and that management should be individual and flexible. Regarding children the report said that there is an increased onset in secondary age children and made the observation that, although there is no cure for CSF/ME, the condition has been found to improve in most patients without intervention. Patients may therefore, it stated, decline treatment; neither the fact of a child having unexplained symptoms, nor the exercising of selective choice about treatment or education, constituted evidence of abuse. Premature pressure to return to education could be particularly damaging. The report commented that children seem to be more vulnerable to the misconception that the illness is all in the mind.

The outcome was bitterly disappointing for the ME groups as there was no understanding that this was really a conflict between two factions regarding research goals and treatment regimes. It was also alarming that as far as children were concerned the report advocated that their illness should be treated by consultant psychiatrists as well as consultant physicians. Their disappointment was compounded when the Medical Research Council (MRC) announced that eight million pounds was to be put towards research into treatment programmes recommended by psychiatrists. The trial was called the PACE trial and was to take place over the next five years.

PACE stands for pacing, graded activity, cognitive behavioural therapy and evaluation. Adaptive pacing is staying within the limits of a finite amount of energy, which may improve symptoms (ie. the patients feel better) but at the expense of disability (ie. they can do less or the same amount of activity). Graded Exercise Therapy (GET) means graded exposure to activity which was previously avoided. Cognitive Behavioural Therapy (CBT) is aimed at changing a patient's beliefs about their illness, so that they focus on how they are feeling, and it helps them to structure rest, sleep, and activity which is gradually increased. The trial was led by P. White, M. Sharpe and Trudie Chalder and it was overseen by Prof. Simon Wesseley. If the trials failed to prove advantageous to the patient then the predictors of poor outcome were pervasive inactivity, concurrent anxiety and depression, current membership of a self-help group and receiving disability benefits. The risks to patients who undertook the trial was that the patients might get worse. (AFME reported that GET and CBT were likely to make patients worse.) The research results were not published, as it transpired, until 2011, seven years later. While this work was in progress no other research or investigation would be funded.

The only serious criticism of the CMO report came from Malcolm Hooper, Emeritus Professor of Medicinal Chemistry at the University of Sunderland, and Sally Montague. They were particularly concerned that clinicians were advised that only limited investigations are necessary. Their other objection was that the report could not be wholly objective since a great many of the papers that supported the findings had been written by members of the working group. Hooper and Montague argued that this did not give evidence of an unbiased report.

When the PACE trial was completed the results were published in *The Lancet*. GET and CBT were endorsed as the treatment of choice and the media reported that patients would need to work harder to get better. Headlines read 'Exercise cures chronic fatigue,' or 'ME sufferers better pushing their limits'. The study claimed that six in ten mild to moderate CFS/ME patients had beneficial results.

Whatever tribulations the ME child has to endure it is the stigma of unbelief that is their greatest burden. Illness can be tolerated if the patient is surrounded by care and compassion. This was an aspect that Dr Speight understood so well when he advised that everyone around the child believed what he had to say. This understanding can be nurtured more easily if the medical establishment, and the media and therefore their readers, would not show such scepticism. At times the press coverage is blatantly critical, and more distressingly, has ridiculed the notion of ME.

Chris may, jokingly, say that he rather approves of the name 'yuppie flu', but only because he has learnt to live with ME. Initially he was not so happy with the label that he wanted his fellow students to be aware that he had had ME. The pervasiveness of the disbelief is apparent by the screeds of literature written in an effort to dispel the stigma, by those who have to cope with the illness. Yet with so many sufferers in the UK, and many more world wide, there has to be a reason why this attitude continues.

What do psychiatrists believe is happening in CFS/ME? In her book, which is aimed at children, Trudie Chalder explained how CFS is understood. She writes that "CFS can start after an illness, or after a stressful time like going to a new school. It is likely that the causes of your CFS will differ from the reasons which keep the illness going Your muscles are weak because you are out of condition. If your muscles are weak the blood collects in your legs and less goes round your brain making you feel dizzy. The more you rest the more fatigued you will feel. When you have had a symptom for a long time it is understandable that you will worry about it. The more you worry the more you notice it and the bigger the problem will become. Each thing affects the others and it is easy to get caught up in a vicious cycle of worsening fatigue and symptoms. If resting has meant that your sleep pattern has changed, your body clock may have been disrupted."

She recommends: sleep, hygiene, setting aside a worry time, having an activity schedule, problem solving for their perfectionist personalities, for facing stressful events, and changing unhelpful thoughts. If children stick to these rules they will begin to feel better and their sleep will improve. On dealing with anxiety she says. "Feeling anxious is part of normal thought and behaviour. The effects on the body of anxiety are headaches, dizziness, blurred vision, hot flushes, dry mouth, choking feeling, fatigue, tension in muscles, breathing difficulties, heart thumping, stomach nausea, pins and needles in arms or legs, urge to go to the toilet, rubbery legs and trembling fingers. These are normal reactions to stress."

The book goes on to diary keeping, pages for changing unhelpful beliefs, pages for grading exercise or increasing activity. "Stick to the plan regardless of how you feel," she advises.

It is difficult to see how an anxiety state which speeds up the body can contribute to fatigue in the brain and in the muscles. Or how resting can cause dizziness. It is curious that so many children, with no prior knowledge and isolated from each other, can show such similar symptoms when there is not an underlying medical condition responsible. It is unlikely that anxiety states are so numerous. At best the explanation and treatment approach offered by psychiatry is innocuous; a formalising of an old-fashioned convalescence of gentle encouragement towards activity alongside compassionate regard for their malaise. At worst it appears to blame the child for their illness because it aims at changing their beliefs about feeling ill. The mind is a powerful machine. How easy it would be to create a problem, in the child's case a guilt complex, that they themselves were perpetuating their disease.

The final and unique form of harm that the psychiatric powers endorse is the persistent recommendation that no investigations, or only limited medical tests, are appropriate.

The fear that diagnosis of ME generates is not only because of the illness itself, but because of an awareness of the powers of the psychiatrists. Unlike other neurological diseases (but in common with meningitis) patients can recover from ME and as a result countless treatments, including psychiatry, claim that they were responsible.

Physical Illness?

"Time is not a good healer
It is an indifferent and perfunctory one."

Dame Ivy Compton-Burnett

It is hardly surprising that the unravelling of ME should be difficult. In the absence of obvious physical features it is not an enticing prospect for any researcher. It is even less of an attractive proposition for any organisation funding research. These organisations, in the absence of government money from the MRC, tend to be pharmaceutical firms. These firms will only be interested if there is the likelihood of drug treatment. No firm is going to invest in a vague label of chronic fatigue syndrome/myalgic encephalomyelitis when no cause had been found and where the syndrome has an assortment of vague signs and symptoms.

When some doctors began to suggest that CFS/ME was perhaps a psychiatric illness, and these illnesses are often treated with drugs, then companies began to be interested.

The factor that favours research into psychiatric illness as opposed to physical or organic illness, is the cost. It costs an enormous amount to run rigorous laboratory trials into medical conditions which may produce no conclusive results. It is relatively cheap to produce papers on psychiatric conditions. It is therefore possible to produce a great many psychiatric papers for the same cost as one medical trial. As a result, in areas where they are interested, psychiatrists can very quickly dominate a subject. This was the case with CFS/ME. As the momentum grew so did the force of the argument that CFS/ME was a case of false illness beliefs and an example of a somatoform disease. In other words, the physical symptoms that the patients were experiencing were due to the state of their mental health.

In contrast ME patients steadfastly maintained that they had a sick body and if they had a mental health problem, which the majority disputed, it was solely due to their having an unexplained physical illness. The two groups became, and still are, entrenched in their views. The physical lobby have neither the money to research nor the strength in numbers to influence policy. The psychiatric lobby hold all the cards in that they have a wealth of research papers to support their views and the weight of the medical profession behind them to implement their programmes.

While the two factions of the medical profession battle this out, each staking their careers on their beliefs, the patients wait, ignored, for a relief for their suffering. The doctors who are not involved in the struggle, in an effort to do the best for their patients and so as to work in line with medical establishment guidelines, are unable to do anything but offer psychiatrically led treatment on the lines of the PACE trial.

It would seem that it was the realisation that there would be no government funding for research into the medical causes of ME for the duration of the PACE trial that galvanised the ME world. Despite the fact that many of the campaigners, support group workers, medical advisers and even the research workers suffered from ME themselves, there was an explosion of activity. By 2002 there were countless local support groups and eight charities dealing with the different aspects of ME. When the numbers of sick people involved are considered this is not surprising. Where it is surprising is those that have recovered from ME do not, on the whole, want to be associated with it. They have lost a massive chunk of their lives to the illness already. In addition, because of the long duration of ME many people lose their jobs and are on a reduced income. There is not the financial base to draw on when facing the realities of fund-raising. Furthermore, although recovered, many people with ME do not have the reserves of energy which are needed for fund-raising activities. However, having said all that, new research pockets were emerging. Each one funded through charities.

In Perth in Scotland ME Research UK was set up which focussed mainly on blood abnormalities. In Glasgow Caledonian University and Glasgow University, research into muscle fatigue and genes began to be developed. At King's College London there was also research into genes. At Essex Centre for Neurological Science Dr Chaudhiri researched into fatigue. In Belgium researchers were looking at exercise and ME. In the USA a new Institute, the Whittemore Peterson Institute in Nevada, was opened purely for neuro-immune diseases, because they were concerned at the lack of available doctors to deal with a growing number of patients with ME/CFS and related illnesses.

Scientists were searching in every system of the body for abnormalities which would give a clue as to what is the cause, or what is happening in ME. At the very least their search is to find a consistent test that could be a diagnostic marker for the illness. In the circulatory system they looked for abnormalities in the lining of the blood vessels which is called the endothelium. If this lining is healthy then a chemical, acetylcholine, can regulate blood vessels to dilate if the person is hot, or to contract if the person is cold. Scientists have noticed that the blood vessels of ME patients, unlike healthy patients or those with blood pressure problems, dilated for longer. They believe that this is due to acetylcholine, which dilates blood vessels, not being removed quickly enough. They have also found this substance in patients' muscles and nerves. Investigations were conducted into whether the increase in acetylcholine in the blood could be measured and then be used as a diagnostic test. A interesting factor was discovered when the scientists did various tests on two different substances that make blood vessels dilate or contract. ME patients reacted differently to other patient control groups, and it was a reaction that was normally found in people who do physical training. There is an argument here to explain why exercise might harm ME patients. If their blood is already overreacting, then exercise might increase that reaction, and could be detrimental.

Apoptosis is the word used for cell death. Cells are being produced and are dying off all the time in the body but they do it in a regulated fashion. Scientists looked at the rate of cell death of the neutrophils in the blood and found that they were dying at an increased rate. This happens when patients have an infection. Scientists showed that CFS patients had more dying neutrophils than healthy controls. They also showed in these samples of blood that CFS patients had more debris in the blood that needed to be cleared. Alongside this there was an increase in a factor that encourages new neutrophils to replace the dying ones. When this situation is seen then a chronic inflammatory process and an underlying abnormality of the immune system is suspected.

Regulation of blood volume is also seen to be disturbed in ME. Patients suffer from light-headedness, fluid balance dysfunctions, feeling faint when they stand up, or just feeling awful until they sit or lie down. Their legs and feet, especially in the morning, look blue.

This is called postural orthostatic intolerance (POTS). Just standing up can trigger many of the ME symptoms and the person is not aware of it. They feel nauseous, have altered vision, fatigue, 'brain fog', headache, sweating and pallor. Most teenagers with ME suffer from POTS. This can be tested on a tilt table where the heart rate and blood pressure will increase.

In another study, it was found that ME patients did not have a large enough volume of blood. If they were injected with enough saline to increase the amount of blood circulating then the patients felt better for twenty-four hours.

Endorsing this research, in an oblique fashion, was a statement by the Under-Secretary of State for Health who announced that people with CFS/ME were not able to give blood until they have fully recovered. She said that as the causes for CFS/ME are not understood, people with the condition are deferred from giving blood as a precautionary measure, to protect the safety of the blood supply for patients.

A feature of blood irregularity found in ME patients is oxidative stress. Scientists have found excessive free radicals generated in the blood, urine and muscle of ME patients. Free radicals, molecules which can damage human cells including brain cells, form naturally whenever the body metabolises oxygen and the damage is called oxidative stress. Oxidative stress is associated with lung damage in ME patients. In his book, 'Explaining Unexplained Illnesses', Martin L Pall relates how disturbances to the oxygen cycle at cell level could account for the disease mechanism behind a number of illnesses, including ME.

Central fatigue is a common symptom of neurological diseases which involve the brain and nervous system. This sort of fatigue is quite different from the tiredness that is caused in muscles due to exertion. There are three areas where the fatigue that is experienced by ME patients is centrally mediated. Patients have delayed motor conduction of the nerves to the muscles, similar to that found in Multiple Sclerosis. Patients have delays in the system which controls the activation of muscles. They have an increased perception of effort and have to work harder to achieve a certain result. Patients are unable to activate their muscles fully, although their muscles are normal and there is no evidence to show that the muscles themselves are damaged.

Studies on the brain show loss of vital chemicals such as choline, a loss of volume as if the brain shrinks, and a loss of an adequate blood supply, or blood perfusion, of brain tissue. Work on fatigue and the basal ganglia in the brain was being done by Dr Chaudhiri. Central fatigue may be due to disruption of the systems controlled by the basal ganglia which is particularly sensitive to lack of oxygen and to viruses.

Viruses have been the focus of much attention. Andrew Lloyd of the University of New South Wales monitored thirty-nine newly diagnosed patients with glandular fever. Six months later eight were suffering from chronic fatigue, while the others had no lasting effects. Lloyd suggested that indirect brain injury caused by viral infection might be to blame. Microglial cells, part of the brain's immune system are known to be activated by viral infection. This could result in temporary changes to the brain's pain (and other) pathways.

Entero-viruses have shown to have a high rate of incidences in ME patients. These viruses can cause meningitis and severe throat infections, but they also cause inflammation or degeneration of heart or brain tissue. Some also attack the muscles of the chest wall, bronchi and pancreas. On autopsy ME suicide patients have shown to have active enteroviruses in their brains.

The herpes virus is another found on autopsy. The herpes virus hides dormant away from the immune system in the cells of the nervous system. When the virus is activated or has an outbreak the virus in the nerve cell is transported via the nerves' network. *Herpes simplex* is best known as 'cold sore'. Another herpes virus is *herpes zoster* or 'shingles' which develops from the dormant 'chicken pox' varicella virus. Symptoms of the first infection with herpes simplex virus are usually more severe than subsequent attacks because the body has not had the chance to produce antibodies. The first outbreak of oral herpes or cold sores carries the risk of developing aseptic meningitis. There is no test for aseptic meningitis. Scientists are exploring the possibility of a similar mechanism occurring in ME.

4.2.00 ~~Travaux ... EAST tense~~

Plus ~~Aubergers...Confortin~~

1. Est-ce que tu as mangé à la cantine hier?
   0. Non, j'ai mangé mes sandwiths aux sardines.
2. Qu'est-ce que tu as fait hier après-midi?
   F. Hier après-midi, j'ai vu le médecin.
3. Qu'est-ce que le médecin a fait?
   B. Il m'a envoyé à l'hôpital.
4. Où as-tu passé la nuit?

Homework jotter. 4.2.00

Speaking Test.

Next weekend. Prochain weekend ~~&~~ j'irais avec ~~deux~~ amis à la maison ~~chez~~ moi. Nous jouerons au tennis et le golf. ~~Nous~~ avons neuf trous près de la maison. Nous ferons une feu de joie, et cuit le saucisson. ~~████~~

Short Film :   A last piece of school work   12.12.00

Photography : bullet comes out a gun but everything stops + the camera continues to go forward + into the guys brain — has a flash back of his life etc. then the camera goes back round to the bullit — everything speeds up.

1.6.01 Chris' attempt at writing-note rapid deterioration of writing and spelling.

. I NEEDED TO GET BACK INTO THE HABIT OF WRITING SO THATS WHY I DID THIS. ALL EVENT INCLUDED IN THE ABOVE PAGE ARE TRUE OR BASED ON FUTURE EVENTS. ANY CHARACTERS WHO HAVE ANY SIMILARITIES TO REAL (ALIVE (DEAD) PERSONS IS TOTALLY ON PERPOUSE AND THEY HAVE GIVEN THEIR PERMSION TO APPER IN THE BREAKFAST TIMES. I'D LIKE TO THANK THE BIC™ MEDIUM ROLLERBALL BIRO PEN, WITHOUT WHICH THIS WOULD

3.7.03 Two years later. About to return to school.

Psychiatric Condition?

"He that will not apply new remedies must expect new evils, for time is the great innovator."

Francis Bacon

Parallel to the story of ME, as observed and researched by the physicians, ran that of ME as understood and treated by the psychiatrists. What is puzzling is how this tragic state of affairs came into being.

The concept of a healthy mind in a healthy body, or the interdependence of the two facets of health, does not unfortunately extend into the realm of the health service. Although doctors understand the interaction of the mind and the body, patients are allocated to one discipline or the other. That is how our Health Service is set up. Doctors become either physicians or surgeons and work in physical medicine, or psychiatrists and work in mental health. In the physical world mental health is of secondary, although growing, importance. It is rare that in a psychiatric department there will be extensive physical investigations.

There is, whether we like it or not, a prevailing tendency to place unexplained illnesses under psychiatry. There is a need for everyone who is ill to have a diagnosis, even although this is an unrealistic goal. This is partly so that people can obtain benefits in order that they can live while they are unwell. Chronic Fatigue Syndrome is a useful label for some of these unexplained fatigue states. As no tests as yet can prove that CFS/ME is an organic disease, it becomes reasonable to assume that it could be a mental condition.

In 1986 Dr Melvin Ramsay thought that the scepticism towards ME was beginning to recede. These seeds of doubt had been the result of an interest taken by McEvedy who had made a study of mass hysteria. In early 1970s McEvedy made a study of two outbreaks of mass hysteria and one of overbreathing that had taken place in schools. McEvedy then decided to do a PhD in the same vein.

McEvedy and Beard, who were part of the department of Psychological Medicine at the Middlesex Hospital, asked permission to peruse the records of the nurses involved in the 1955 Royal Free hospital outbreak. Only one person, a Dr Helen Dinsdale had a premonition. "I think it is very possible that you will live to rue the day when you made yourself party to that decision," she told Dr Ramsay. However, permission was granted, and the study, which was designed to determine a possible predisposition to psychoneurosis in the nurses in this affected group, went ahead. In their first paper McEvedy and Beard gave their reasons for regarding the disease at the Royal Free Hospital as a case of mass hysteria. In the second paper they argued that the fourteen outbreaks reviewed by Acheson (in 1959) contained features which justified a similar conclusion but with provisos regarding a few of those outbreaks.

The reaction to this retrospective appraisal was extraordinary. The BMJ congratulated the authors on their paper, tempering it with a guarded warning against placing too much emphasis on appraisals so late after the event. But the damage was done. The story of mass hysteria as a reason for the Royal Free disease was carried by newspapers and even more significantly by *Time* magazine. Some years later the devastating effect of this paper was experienced by Dr Ramsay himself, when trying to explain the aetiology and pathology of ME to colleagues. He found himself silenced by the comment, "but that was long ago proved to be a case of mass hysteria."

From these early rumblings of a possible psychiatric element among the nurses who suffered in the Royal Free outbreak, the diagnosis of ME as a physical disease was questioned, and an increasing number of psychiatrists became interested.

The idea of physical symptoms manifesting themselves as the result of a disturbed mental condition is not a new concept. It was acknowledged that most cases of ME began with an infection, but views became divided as to why the patient did not get better. ME patients believe that they have an ongoing infection which has made changes in their bodies preventing full recovery. Psychiatrists believe that the person's own mental health is preventing this recovery. The critical moment in this shift of emphasis was the Lake Tahoe epidemic, and the subsequent introduction of the term CFS. It was this belief in the power of the mind to heal the body that drove the psychiatrists. They believed that this system was disrupted in all conditions that were now placed under the umbrella term CFS. In the absence of a cause for ME, this benign approach, although unacceptable to ME patients, would have been tolerated. However as more psychiatrists became interested their theories proliferated, and some were prepared to prove that ME was indeed all in the mind. It was only a step for matters to progress to covertly, and occasionally overtly, to accuse mothers of delaying their child's recovery for some psychological reason of their own and to suggest that ME is in fact a result of MSBP or FII (Fabricated or induced illness, the preferred term for Münchausen syndrome by proxy in the UK.) Ean Proctor was the first recorded case.

In 1986, the year when Dr Ramsay, wrote that "victims should no longer have to dread the verdict that 'all your tests are normal, therefore there is nothing wrong with you,'" Ean Proctor fell ill with Post Viral Fatigue Syndrome. During 1987 he became increasingly physically unwell, was unable to speak, was partially paralysed and was developing mental and physical fatigue. His parents finally managed to be referred from the Isle of Man to see a consultant in London where he was diagnosed with Myalgic Encephalitis. In April the next year they went for a return appointment. A registrar in Psychiatry, Dr Simon Wessely, together with Dr Lusk and Dr Turk, took an interest in the case. Dr Lusk wanted to initiate a psychiatric programme of graded exercise with family therapy. Other doctors wanted to admit him to a closed ward. The parents could not afford to stay in London and returned home. Two months later Dr Wessely suggested to the principal social worker on the case that 'the boy was needing a long period of rehabilitation and skilled separation from his parents.' The boy was then removed from his parents by social workers accompanied by police officers. The inference was that the parents were to blame for having imposed 'false illness beliefs' upon him. Convinced that the boy was school-phobic, that he suffered from 'elective mutism' and had 'false illness beliefs' imposed on him by his parents, he was put in a swimming-pool - where he sank to the bottom of the pool since he could not use his arms - to 'shock' him into behaving normally. He was taken to a Fair Ground where doctors thought a ride on a ghost train would force him to cry out and to prove that he could speak. The boy did not come out of the hospital until six months later when his parents found a physician who would treat him. The parents realised that they were the victims of a serious disagreement between two factions of the medical profession. The Isle of Man Parliament, the Tynwald, decision in 1989 entirely vindicated the parents. Unfortunately, in 1992, the McManus Inquiry reversed the decision saying that the parents had brought everything on themselves, and the findings were a substantial victory for the psychiatric lobby. The tragic events cost the family dear. They were forced to leave their home, because of the cruel behaviour of neighbours who assumed from the proceedings that the parents had been abusing their son.

The psychiatrists involved in his case were also involved with the 1996 Royal Colleges report on CFS/ME who maintain that CFS/ME should be placed under a mental health category. Since 1986 until the present day ME children and their families have continually found themselves under suspicion of having MSBP. Some have had their children removed.

Until a definitive test can be found to prove otherwise there seems no reason for this to stop. The belief is so strong, in some cases, that the child will be harmed by being left in the family home, that doctors will go to great lengths to protect the child.

A young girl from Chalfont St. Giles became unwell in 1996 and was diagnosed with ME when she was twelve. A year later her consultant, Dr Cheetham, believing she needed hospitalisation, physiotherapy and psychiatric treatment, suggested that she had been emotionally abused. Her father was devastated. "It is very difficult for a family with a sick child to feel that they are being accused of causing her illness." They went to Dr Speight for a second opinion. Dr Cheetham disagreed with her treatment and obtained her medical notes without consent and continued to interfere for two years, despite the family having transferred to another specialist. The GMC found that Dr Cheetham's behaviour had been unacceptable. Even the social services called by Dr Cheetham's colleagues decided that the girl was not at risk. However when the case was reviewed on appeal the GMC cleared the Consultant stating that they could not be sure that this was a case of serious professional misconduct.

If a diagnosis of MSBP is unfounded the prospects for the child and family are terrifying. It is this fear, more then any other, that makes the unravelling of ME so vital. It is frustrating to ME patients that this aspect of ME is not understood, and that open debate and further research into the cause of ME is not forthcoming. Psychiatrists who believe that there is nothing organically wrong with the patients see no reason for this dialogue or for such research.

The signs and symptoms of ME are similar, in many aspects, to those of anxiety states. For this reason psychiatrists feel that their views are justified. There are a myriad of papers that have been published which endorse this view. Moreover the PACE trial has proved successful, they feel, and the psychiatrists' current view has been endorsed. Patients will recover and expensive treatment into an organic cause can be avoided.

Unfortunately the PACE trial which at best appears to be helpful and at worst innocuous, can have a different perspective. ME patients see recent events as dangerous and threatening. Dangerous because ME patients may well become worse from following advice, and threatening because if they do not follow advice then their children may be removed. They do not have sufficient evidence to convince sceptics that they are not over-reacting.

To the uninitiated the rationale behind the PACE trial appears logical and warranted. If ME is detached from CFS these approaches and a trial into them is a reasonable solution. If ME is considered an organic illness, then it is possible to understand the antagonism towards the trials. Firstly, should ME be proved to have a medically explained cause, the nine years since the report was launched until the result of the PACE trial was published, will have been wasted. During this time medical research could have taken place, but it was put on hold. Secondly, if ME patients are correct and exercise does make them worse, the treatment regime now advocated will cause more rather than fewer patients to be ill. Thirdly, CBT has been used, with children as well as with adults, to change illness beliefs. If the children are ill with an organic disease, then CBT causes unnecessary feelings of guilt that they are the cause of their illness, and encourages them to attempt things that they have instinctively avoided. Fourthly, now that the medical establishment has been instructed through the PACE trial and NICE guidelines how to treat ME patients, anyone who queries it is likely to set themselves up for trouble.

Dr Sarah Myhill was suspended by the GMC in 2010 for eighteen months for using investigative procedures and alternative medicine approaches to cases of ME, allergies and other non-specific diagnoses.

Dr Nigel Speight had an eighteen month investigation by the GMC. He started to be harassed in 2003 for political reasons within his Trust but his work in ME was one of the instruments that they chose to use against him. He got the feeling that any complaint against him would be listened to. In 2009 a child psychiatrist wrote to the Trust accusing him of overdiagnosing the condition. He was accused also of keeping children off school unnecessarily and confining them to bed for long periods. His Medical Director referred him to the National Clinical Assessment Centre where, despite being of retirement age, he had to undergo a clinical assessment including a three hour written examination, which he passed in the top three per cent.

The established consensus of what constitutes CFS includes ME. Experts in CFS advise the General Medical Council (GMC), the government, the armed forces, the insurance firms and direct benefit agencies. One of the most tangible effects of a CFS label for a ME patient is on their financial situation. CFS is a nebulous diagnosis and carries little weight when patients are trying to access benefits or claim on insurance. If ME was recognised as a separate illness, their medical assessments and consequent financial allowances would not entail the degree of doubt and uncertainty that they now carry.

In 2002 in Dumfries and Galloway a mother with ME was refused benefits. She had a fourteen year old daughter to support and in despair she committed suicide. In some cases suicide can be caused by despair with the illness itself.

In 2010 Kay Gilderdale was remanded in custody on bail charged with the attempted murder of her daughter. The thirty-one year old Lynn had become ill after a BCG vaccination and she was diagnosed with ME, aged fourteen, after suffering from bronchitis, tonsillitis and glandular fever. Advice from her GP had been to encourage Lynn to take as much exercise as possible, which proved to be the worst course of action. 'It got to a point where she was totally bed-ridden.' She was unable to walk, talk or drink. Lynn had a seventeen-year battle with ME, enduring constant pain and requiring twenty-four hour care. Lynn kept an on-line journal. She wrote: "Imagine having the bones of a hundred-year-old woman, unable to move without risking a fracture. Imagine being unable to get the spinning thoughts out of your head, other than by slowly typing emails ... I have nothing left and I am spent ... It's going to be my time to go very soon."

Meanwhile patients will continue to go to the doctor to say that they cannot get well and that they cannot do the things that they want to do. They will be prescribed GET. They will be prescribed, albeit in a graded fashion, the very thing that they have gone to the doctor to obtain help with. It is understandable that they are confused and feel let down by the medical profession.

The kindest interpretation of GET and CBT is that a patient is guided and nurtured to a careful return to health and activity and is gently dealt with through the natural ups and downs and frustrations of a very slow recovery from a mysterious and horrid illness. This could as easily be described as a period of convalescence. If the natural course of ME is four and a half years then a greater part of the time must be taken up by convalescence. GET and CBT could be described therefore as professionally supervised convalescence. The Mothers of ME children have come to that conclusion unaided. The CMO report says that children tend to recover without intervention.

What happened to derail a disease that was on the way to being recognised? What happened to fuel an alternative approach that has gained momentum ever since? How was it that such a devastating disease, which at times becomes highly contagious and presents as epidemics, and which was recognised across the world, underwent such a change in the opinion of professionals? For fifteen or so years after the outbreak of the Royal Free disease in 1955 the recognition and description of ME by Dr Melvin Ramsay had been accepted by the medical profession. There had been no disputing the reality of Myalgic Encephalomyelitis as a physiological disease until the end of the sixties.

One doctor in Canada decided to investigate how this radical shift in the perception of ME had come about. Dr Byron Hyde was a junior doctor at the time of the Lake Tahoe epidemic in 1984 and attended the subsequent inquiry in 1987. He watched as the Lake Tahoe epidemic was explained away as one of the Epstein-Barr virus (glandular fever) despite glaring facts to prove to the contrary. The virus causing the epidemic had a fast incubation period of approximately a week, whereas glandular fever has an incubation span of forty days. He witnessed the interest of psychiatrists at the inquiry and saw the emergence of a new category of disease, namely CFS.

By 1992 Dr Hyde had become increasingly involved in examining cases of CFS/ME. He was able, within this umbrella label of CFS, to give alternative diagnoses to a number of cases which included some missed diagnoses of rare or fatal diseases. He also sifted out over 2,000 unmistakable cases of ME. That year he became part of a large body of doctors to collate the most extensive collection of known scientific facts about ME. This became known as the Nightingale Foundation, because Florence Nightingale is believed to have suffered from ME.

Dr Hyde began his quest to find out the truth behind the 1970 papers of McEvedy and Beard by travelling to Los Angeles to interview doctors and nurses affected by that outbreak. This was one of the outbreaks that McEvedy in his second paper had attributed, by extension of his hypothesis, with being a case of mass hysteria. He met many of those affected and found that some still carried evidence of the disease.

Dr Hyde sought out Dr Ramsay and interviewed him. Dr Ramsay explained that Dr McEvedy had never examined any of the patients whose records were held by the Royal Free, nor had he interviewed them. Furthermore he had never interviewed Dr Ramsay or any of his colleagues who had attended the patients with ME and who together had written the original account which had been published in the BMJ. Again, many of those affected by the Royal Free Disease were still suffering. It became apparent that it was a common practice with psychiatrists not to undertake a physical examination of their patients. In a case in 1989, before Justice Macpherson, the lawyer Mr Beckman, who was representing a patient, asked if Dr Beard himself had examined the patient. Dr Beard replied that a psychiatrist does not normally do a physical examination.

To ascertain for himself the sources of the original papers published by McEvedy, Dr Hyde sought out the schools where the mass hysteria and over-breathing had occurred. He was able to find the headmistress of one of the schools. Even though it was years since the McEvedy incident she was still quite angry with him. She recalled the incident in great detail. She said that Dr McEvedy had never been to the school, had never examined any of the children, and that his thesis was a work of total imagination. She said that the girls did not suffer from mass hyperventilation but had been ill with a self-limiting gastro-enteritis that, depending on the pupil, had lasted for one to three days and consisted primarily of nausea and explosive diarrhoea. There was no mass hysteria.

No-one when accepting the paper at the University had thought to verify the acts behind the thesis.

There was one final logical path for Dr Hyde to follow which was to find and question Dr McEvedy in person. Dr McEvedy said that he was happy to see him. "Dr McEvedy was now a widower and lived in a small house in a west-end of London suburb in a shambolic disarray of books, bags, odds and ends, and papers. He had pursued his career as a psychiatrist but was above all a historian." (By 2005 he had published the Penguin Atlas of almost every history of every continent.) He was a brilliant man and cordial, and in other circumstances Dr Hyde would have been comfortable in his company. He asked him about the cases concerning the two schools and particularly if he had any records concerning his visits? Dr McEvedy said he did not. Dr Hyde then asked why had he written up the Free Hospital epidemic as hysteria without any careful exploration of the basis of the thesis. Dr McEvedy replied that it was an easy PhD, and so why not? Dr Hyde said that he hoped that he had changed his mind about the hysterical basis of Myalgic Encephalitis but asked him if he was of the same impression. Dr McEvedy answered that, 'Of course he was of the same impression. They were just a group of hysterical people.' Finally Dr Hyde asked Dr McEvedy why he did his PhD on the Royal Free. Dr McEvedy again replied that, 'It was an easy PhD. Why not?'

Dr McEvedy died in 2005. Dr Ramsay's views of McEvedy were confirmed. There was no medical basis for any of Dr McEvedy's statements.

The consequences of a psychiatric approach to an organic disease can be that the patient is not seeking a solution to a psychiatric problem, therefore they will be reluctant to co-operate when psychiatric treatment is offered. Patients may have to adhere to treatment regimes which have the potential to cause harm. Drugs used for the treatment of psychogenic disorders may be used and these are known to react badly in patients with ME. Finally, by refusing psychiatric treatment, psychiatrists claim that this is yet a further aspect of their Irrational Illness Perception (IIP). This gives the psychiatrists dealing with ME *carte blanche* to determine as mentally ill any parent or child who refuses the psychiatric aetiology. They have named this disorder Persistent Refusal Syndrome (PRS) and that contributing to this condition can be sexual abuse or domestic violence and that it is potentially life-threatening.

This last section gives the right to the doctor to force-feed children, use physical restraints, section (admit to psychiatric hospital) and to team up with teachers and social workers for a 'tough love' policy. The most serious and fraudulent consequences of refusal by families and patients to accept the psychiatric aetiology of ME is that of MSBP. Moreover, a unique form of harm to sufferers is the persistent recommendation from the leading group of psychiatrists that no investigations, or only limited medical tests, are appropriate or necessary.

The cruelty that these psychiatric powers endorse is the single most distressing consequence of a psychiatric label for ME. Accounts abound of management of ME that disgrace the 20th and 21st century. You only have to read *Shattered* by Lynn Mitchell, *The Dossier of Shame* by the Tymes Trust, or Ean Proctor's or Sophia Mirza's stories to see a few. In a questionnaire put out by the Tymes Trust four per cent of parents had been branded with the condition MSBP. National Statistics show that it affects just one in ten thousand families, 'It is incomprehensible that such inhuman strategies are employed in a branch of medicine that professes to heal the mind.' said Per Dalen, a professor of psychiatry in Sweden.

It is twenty-five years, the age that Chris is now, since the advent of psychiatric control of ME. Their hold is as strong as ever. ME patients believe that their illness is physical and research results from around the world are bearing this out. Dr Melvin Ramsay and all those who studied and were involved with the outbreaks of ME believed that it was a physical illness. Someone said that ME is here to challenge the twenty-first century. Perhaps it is only with emerging technology that this complex disease will be unravelled. It is salutary to think that this disease has already been under investigation for almost seventy-five years.

Postscript

There is evidence that reaching the age of sixteen no longer removes the fear of a young person being removed from their home. Dr Speight looked after Tim Hartley from the age of thirteen. He diagnosed ME. Four months after Dr Speight retired, the new Consultant moved against the family. The High Court ruled that Timothy Hartley lacked the capacity to have a say in his own life decisions. The recommendation was that he should be removed from his mother's care and placed in a Local Authority Hostel on a long term basis. His mother's access to him should be restricted and supervised. Timothy Hartley was twenty-two years old. The professionals treated this as a case of MSBP or FII without explicitly saying so, which made it hard to counter. The medical profession are using the Mental Incapacity Act to remove those over sixteen who they believe are victims of MSBP.

Timothy Hartley was placed in a SSD (Social Services Department) hostel with a myriad of carers which caused him more frequent fits. Timothy's Mother was threatened with jail if she did not hand over his savings to the SSD. She told Dr Speight that she felt like going to jail to bring the case in to the open.

Of the young people who have ME with whom we are acquainted, only half have recovered. Two girls and one boy at Chris' school in Ayrshire contracted ME. Emma, from the station episode, has trained to be a vet but the other two have not recovered. Alice's older son is working full time and her daughter is on the mend after contracting ME in 2007 at the age of sixteen. Jane's son Hamish contracted ME in 2006 and was unable to work for four years. He is now working part time. He was a highly employable computer expert, and a fit mountaineer prior to his illness. Davina is still housebound with no signs of recovery. Nicholas is ambulant but his brain fog still stifles his creative talent.

It took a long while before Chris' ability to make decisions returned. Any form of mental multi-tasking required an inordinate amount of effort and I would be called upon to arrange the repair of a malfunctioning computer or give advice with his budgeting. He was twenty-one before he was ready to take his driving test. Chris passed first time which gave him some satisfaction, as both his brothers had needed two re-sits. Leading up to his final year dissertation matters came to a head as he verged on a relapse. It is not unusual for students to have problems at this time and we told Chris to come home. He struggled daily, but this was one of his last episodes, and there have been only minor dips since.

Chris secured a job the week after he left University. With his life now settled and into a routine, he took a few days off and came home. He and I were in the kitchen one evening and he chatted to me as I prepared supper.

"Chris," I plunged in. "I need to publish this book." I did not need to remind him that a girl had died of ME, he already knew, although I had not elaborated on the details.

"I know." he replied with a seriousness that I was not expecting.

"So?" I asked, "Will you give me permission?"

He gave me a look, but I knew that this time he did.

The years that Chris struggled with ME are now pigeon-holed. He has walked away from that person to emerge whole, confident and with an inspiring sense of proportion. "They have the edge over us", commented the father of a teenager who had had a similar history of ME. "They have faced the abyss and returned." These young people never treat life lightly. They adopt a work ethic, a consideration for others, a non-judgemental approach and grasp every opportunity. This seems to be the hallmark of those who emerge having recovered. It is a worthwhile and remarkable legacy, but the price that they have paid has been the loss of their childhood.

Once Chris recovered it was tempting to avoid any further connection with ME, but two aspects of this experience prevented me. There are still very many young people suffering daily, some known to me personally, who require someone to fight on their behalf. They need recognition that they are ill, help while they are ill, compassion and understanding, treatment or a cure, and they need reassurance that they are not under threat of being removed from their homes. They are too unwell, and their carers too absorbed, to do this for themselves.

Secondly, ME has a known course of relapses and remissions. No one who has had ME is ever immune from the possibility of a relapse. This spectre is never completely vanquished and Chris and I are still unwillingly enmeshed in this disease.

A great number of people have already raised awareness and contributed towards research or support services using a variety of fund-raising activities. In response to the questions that I have been asked over the past twelve years on the subject of ME, and to present the case for the victims of this tragically debilitating disease, I decided to write "What Is Wrong With ME".

Others' Stories

1

Recovery after twenty years of a girl who contracted ME while at University

Our daughter fell ill in her second year at University. At first it seemed like a recurring flu bug and during the early part of 1987 she would return home from her hall of residence as she did not feel well enough to go to lectures. Soon these periods at home became more and more frequent, until it became obvious that she would have to give up her university life.

She developed a range of frightening symptoms - a profound weakness which meant that she could not get out of bed, continuous head pain, sensitivity to noise and light, involuntary ticks and tremors. These were constant but others came and went - sometimes she slept for hours, other times insomnia was a feature. Obviously, she had been back and forward to the GP and eventually a consultant told her she had ME. His prognosis was that it might take a year until she would be able to resume life - a rueful prospect but, in retrospect, how lucky that would have been.

Days, months, years went by. Family life went on as best it could but C was still very ill. She could only tolerate visits from friends for minutes, she could not watch TV and even having a bath exhausted her. The GP visited on a regular basis but could offer no real treatment, although she was willing to try anything we suggested as a possible help. Desperation drove us to seek 'cures' from unconventional sources - homeopathy, osteopathy, and some less reputable avenues. It was the investment of hope that was the worst, not so much the loss of money.

After three years a spell in hospital seemed to lead to a very gradual turnaround. C learned how to manage her symptoms and, although not completely recovered, she was able to go back to University on a part-time basis and finish her degree.

Unfortunately this partial recovery was short-lived. She became bed-bound again, with an acceleration of her old symptoms, and periodic depression. Her life was passing in a blur of pain, exhaustion and hopelessness.

Other members of our family coped in various ways. My husband chose not to read anything about the illness, it being too painful. I joined support groups and campaigned for greater recognition leading to better treatment. I was a member of the Cross-Party group set up in the Scottish Parliament where I met other sufferers and parents and found this to be therapeutic.

An article in the press led to a therapist, with a new-found way of dealing with ME, ringing C and offering her help. C decided to try Mickel therapy as she had heard some good outcomes from it. Almost from the start she began to make gradual progress and around a year later she was well enough to move in with her partner. They now have two little children. Over the twenty years of C's illness I have always believed it to be purely bio-medical and C's turnaround would seem to cast some doubt on this. I still believe that Mickel Therapy may not have worked in the early stages but I am grateful for it and especially to the therapist who affected the change.

2

Recovery of a twenty-one year old girl.

I first became ill in 1996 when I was five years old. It started like so many cases of ME with a viral infection. I had a sore throat, nausea, stomach pains, all on top of what seemed to be the ever present tiredness. It was as if I had new symptoms every day. Literally overnight I turned from a very active little girl who loved to dance into someone who could not make it through a morning of school.

Despite the fact that I was practically a text book study of ME in children, the doctors I went to see all seemed resolutely determined not to diagnose me and indeed were very determined that I was making it up. Luckily I had parents who believed me and a mother with a veterinary degree who knew exactly what I had, a certainty finally backed up by Dr Nigel Speight, who gave me an official diagnosis.

I was ill for thirteen years. Never bedridden but often housebound for many months at a time. The state of my health fluctuated over the years so that I could sometimes do things (mostly bouts of concentrated schoolwork) and more often not. After many years it got to the point where I could not even remember what it was like not to be in pain.

Through the long (interminable) years my family and I tried many things to try and help me get better. To list them all would take many pages, and whilst some helped for a little while or seemed to treat some of the symptoms nothing actually got me to the point of what you would call health. Until I went on a course and did the Lightning Process.

I had heard about it a few years before I actually did it. (I was trying other things and in ME circles you are always hearing about something.) After pretty much collapsing at the end of my first year at University I had nothing to lose.

Whilst I was naturally sceptical about the amazing testimonials, statistics, first hand accounts, etc., I was determined to go in with an open mind.

Within days of doing the Lightning Process my health improved dramatically. I went on holiday with my family, I could walk around town — most importantly I had times without pain. Within a month I had got my first ever job — waitressing of all things! Since doing the Lightning Process (and continue to do it as it's an on-going process) my health has changed completely for the better. My second year at University was better then easy, it was fun! I was able to do normal things which everyone else takes for granted — cooking for myself, shopping, studying hard all the year round.

After a few months I began to feel comfortable referring to my ME in the past tense believing that I would continue to feel well day after day. Best of all I get to enjoy life without constant physical pain and exhaustion, get up each day knowing I can do anything a healthy person can do, as I am one.

3

A twenty-eight year old who has not recovered.

Nicholas has the classic ME bloodless and pale face, forearms and hands. He is slight of build and his right leg has muscle spasm rigidity. After University he travelled in USA but since then has had to live at home. His brain fog is so crippling that it stifles his creativity and is a severe handicap when communicating in interviews, on the telephone, or even writing. He suffers from sleep reversal and is socially isolated except for acquaintances made via the internet.

(Note the brevity with which he has typed his ME account to reduce the effort that was required)

1. A bad case of flu at the end of term 1 secondary school led to two years in bed.

2. Psychiatrists put me into a special school. rape victims/mental abuse victims/physical abuse victims/violent teenagers. Managed to get out after two days. Was threatened by a nurse that I could be taken away from my parents.

3. Was put back into secondary education but was constantly too ill to be there and got taken home 80% of the time.

4. By the time I reached sixteen I was told by a kind English teacher that I didn't have to be there and it was legal for me to leave.

5. Went to art college for six years. Health was much much better but would still sweat abnormal amounts.

6. Came back to live with my parents and gradually got worse again.

7. Severely reduced exercise helps enormously. With normal life exercise I unfortunately get very, very ill. People do not understand this. Stress seems to make things a lot worse, so I try to avoid stressful scenarios. Still sweat abnormal amounts. and find myself getting frights very, very easily.

4

The recovery of a thirty-four year old girl.

I have to start this piece about my recovery by saying that I was ill for over fifteen years and tried many conventional and unconventional treatments with no success. I understand and feel for everyone who is still ill and hasn't yet found his or her path to wellness.

My recovery very definitely started with a visit to see a doctor in Dublin four years ago. I found Dr Magovern after reading Dr Teitelbahm's book *Fatigue to Fantastic*. His protocol seemed to leave no stone uncovered and treated aggressively two of my worst symptoms - lack of quality sleep and high levels of pain in my muscles and my joints.

Dr Teitelbaum lives in Maryland, USA, so a trip there was out of the question. I looked on his website to see if there were any doctors in UK following his protocol. The nearest was Dr Patrick Magovern in Dublin, Ireland. He had been on one of Dr Teitelbaum's courses.

Dr Magovern is a conventionally trained GP who practises using 'Integrative Medicine'. His approach really appealed to me. He used any conventional medicines deemed necessary and, in conjunction, looked at all other aspects of health, using nutrition, vitamins, herbs and homeopathic medicine to give the patient the best chance of recovery. He even talked about finding out about a patient's passions in life. I remember him saying several times he wanted to see me back horse riding again.

After a long consultation I went to a hospital in Dublin and had what seemed like an endless amount of blood taken. I was given medication that dramatically improved the quality of my sleep. I was also given vitamins, minerals and several different amino acids.

I had dramatic improvements in my pain levels following lidnocaine and 'Myers' IV infusion in Dr Magovern's surgery but this was fairly short lived. Although Dr Magovern found many abnormalities in my blood tests, the most significant discovery was a gut parasite called blastosis hominis. An initial course of antibiotics gave me a seemingly miraculous improvement in my joint pain. My father will never forget me getting out of the car and walking down the street without my wheelchair when I was on the antibiotic treatment. Unfortunately, the antibiotics didn't kill the parasite, my symptoms returned, and we had to think about what to do.

After some Internet research I discovered that a hospital in Australia had a triple antibiotic protocol to eradicate the parasite. I discussed this with Dr Magovern and he agreed to fax a prescription to a pharmacy in Australia, as the antibiotics weren't available in the UK. I have to say that the ten days taking this combination of antibiotics were probably some of the worst days of my illness. I was incredibly ill and the treatment left me underweight and extremely weak.

However, my sleep was improving, pain levels were better and I felt there had been a 'shift' in my symptoms. Being in such a weak state I had weekly acupuncture and cranial osteopathy, both of which were incredibly supportive.

I had six months of gradual improvement and now felt well enough to travel to Glasgow for a type of treatment that involved listening to your body's core intelligence and acting on your core emotions, ignoring any 'head-based' thoughts. My practitioner, Lynda Carnochan, had been ill with ME herself and her insight and determination to help her patients is inspirational. In fact I think most people, with or without ME would benefit from learning the skills she taught me!

I had another six months of making amazing progress, learning to drive, going out and about without my wheelchair and getting my life back. I still had severe stomach pains and digestive problems but all in all I felt lucky to be so much better.

Suddenly I then got Glandular Fever and had several months feeling very ill again which was devastating.

Fortunately the locum doctor who saw me during that time noticed that I had a low IGA and that this had been giving false negatives for coeliac disease testing. I now follow a very strict gluten free diet. It has been life changing.

I now look and feel 100% better. My life is great and I feel lucky for every day that I can take my dog for a walk. Feeling tired after a hard days work is so different from the sickening tiredness that I used to suffer from. Many people helped me on my road to recovery and I am thankful for each and every one of them.

References

Acheson, E. D., 'The Clinical Syndrome Variously Called Benign Myalgic Encephomyelitis. Iceland Disease and Epidemic Neuromyasthenia.' *The American Journal of Medicine 26 (4): 569–95.* 1959

Anderson, Rachel, *This Strange New Life.* Oxford University Press, 2006

Chalder, Trudie, *Self-Help for Chronic Fatigue Syndrome.* Blue Stallion Publications, 2002

Chaudhuri, Abhijit and Shepherd, Charles, *ME/CFS/PVFS: An exploration of key clinical issues.* ME Association, 2005

Chief Medical Officers Working Group, 2002. *Report of CFS/ME.* http://www.dh.gov.uk/en/Publicationsandstatistics/Publications/PublicationsPolicyAndGuidance/DH_4064840

Cockshell S.J., Mathias J.L. 'Cognitive functioning in chronic fatigue syndrome: a meta-analysis.' *Psychological Medicine 2010 Aug;40(8):1253-67.*

Ginsberg, Lionel, *Lecture Notes in Neurology.* 9th ed. Wiley-Blackwell, 2010

Goldstein, Jay et al, *Clinical and Scientific Basis of Myalgic Encephalomyelitis/Chronic Fatigue Syndrome.* The Nightingale Research Foundation, 1992

Gregory, Julie, *Sickened: The True Story of a Lost Childhood [A Case History of Münchhausen Syndrome By Proxy]* Random House, 2004

Hyde, Byron, *A Brief History of Myalgic Encephalomyelitis and an irreverent history of CFS.* Presented at Invest In ME London Conference, May 12, 2006.

Hyde, Byron, *Missed Diagnoses: ME and CFS.* Second edition. Lulu, 2011

Jason et al. 'Chronic Fatigue Syndrome: The Need for Subtypes.' *Neuropsychology* March 2005 ME Association Publications.

Klimas N.G., Koneru A.O., 'Chronic Fatigue Syndrome: Inflammation, Immune Function, and Neuroendocrine Interactions.' *Current Rheumatology Reports* 2007, 9:482-487.

ME Research UK *Breakthrough.* Twice yearly.

Pall, Martin, *Explaining 'Unexplained Illnesses'.* Harrington Park Press, 2007

Puri, Basant, *Chronic Fatigue Syndrome: the natural way to treat ME.* Hammersmith Press, 2003.

Ramsay, A. Melvin, *Myalgic Encephalomyelitis and Post Viral Fatigue States. The Saga of Royal Free Disease*. ME Association 1986

Richardson, John, *Enteroviral and Toxic Mediated ME/CFS and other pathologies*. Haworth Medical Press, 1989

Richardson, John, *Myalgic Encephalomyelitis: Guidelines for doctors*. Journal of Chronic Fatigue Syndrome, Vol. 10(1) 2002, pp. 65-80

Twisk, F.N. and Maes, M. 'A review on cognitive behavioural therapy (CBT) and graded exercise therapy (GET) in myalgic encephalitis (ME)/chronic fatigue syndrome (CFS): CBT/GET is not only ineffective and not evidence based, but potentially harmful for many patients with ME/CFS' *Neuroendocrinology Letters* 2009;30(3):284-99.

Tymes Trust, *The Forgotten Children - A Dossier of Shame*. tymestrust.org, 2003

Walker, Martin J., *Skewed: Psychiatric Hegemony and the manufacture of mental illness in Multiple Chemical Sensitivity, Gulf War Syndrome, Myalgic Encephalomyelitis and Chronic Fatigue Syndrome*. Slingshot Publications, 2003

ME, CFS or ME/CFS?
The nomenclature explained

Myalgic Encephalomyelitis (ME) and Chronic Fatigue Syndrome (CFS) or variations of these names are currently used in Britain to describe the condition that is the subject of this book. Because no-one knows exactly what ME/CFS is there is confusion over the name of this illness.

ME is not a recent phenomenon; this name was mainly used until about twenty-five years ago when the new term Chronic Fatigue Syndrome was introduced.

Generally, it is found that people suffering from ME, ME/CFS or CFS prefer the name ME.

The first report of this illness in 1934 called it Epidemic Neuromyasthenia, later reports called it Icelandic disease and another Benign Myalgic Encephalomyelitis (because no-one died). It has also been called Atypical Poliomyelitis and Royal Free Disease. Dr Melvin Ramsay, who reported on a large outbreak in London, settled on Myalgic Encephalomyelitis and this name was accepted for many years. CFS was introduced after an epidemic of a disease with many of the symptoms of ME broke out in 1988 in USA. From then onwards research on these and subsequent patients has been undertaken under this new label, but patients use ME because they do not consider that the broader label reflects the illness which they have.

CFS is an umbrella label for conditions which have not been diagnosed, or where the doctor is unable to give a diagnosis. ME/CFS is used therefore to reflect the more specific symptoms that people with ME suffer.

CFS and ME/CFS are used in research, by the NICE guidelines and by doctors. Where reference to information is drawn from research papers or from information disseminated through self-help Associations, I use CFS and ME/CFS depending on the author. ME is used elsewhere in the narrative because, like other sufferers and their carers, I consider that the label most closely describes the illness that I witnessed.

Useful Contacts

ME Association
7 Apollo Office Court, Radclive Rd, Gawcott, Bucks, MK18 4DF
www.meassociation.org.uk

AYME
Association of Young People with ME
10 Vermont Place, Tongwell, Milton Keynes, MK15 8JA
www.ayme.org.uk

Action for ME
PO Box 2778, Bristol, BS1 9DJ
www.afme.org.uk

Tymes Trust
PO Box 4347, Stock, Ingatestone, CM4 9TE
www.tymestrust.org

25% ME Group
21 Church St., Troon, Ayrshire, KA10 6HT
www.25megroup.org

National ME Centre
Long-term Condition Centre
Gubbins Lane, Harold Wood, Romford, Essex, RM3 0AR
www.nmec.org.uk

Invest in ME
PO Box 561, Eastleigh, Hampshire, SO50 0GQ
www.investinme.org

ME Research UK
The Gateway, North Methven St, Perth, PH1 5PP
www.meresearch.org.uk

Dr Magovern @ www.drummartinclinic.ie

Lightning Source UK Ltd.
Milton Keynes UK
UKOW04f2140230913

217779UK00006B/905/P